Current Controversies in the Approach to Complex Hallux Valgus Deformity Correction

Editor

SUDHEER C. REDDY

FOOT AND ANKLE CLINICS

www.foot.theclinics.com

Consulting Editor
MARK S. MYERSON

March 2020 • Volume 25 • Number 1

ELSEVIER

1600 John F. Kennedy Boulevard • Suite 1800 • Philadelphia, Pennsylvania, 19103-2899

http://www.theclinics.com

FOOT AND ANKLE CLINICS Volume 25, Number 1
March 2020 ISSN 1083-7515, ISBN-978-0-323-69410-0

Editor: Lauren Boyle
Developmental Editor: Nicole Congleton

Foot and Ankle Clinics (ISSN 1083-7515) is published quarterly by Elsevier, Inc., 360 Park Avenue South, New York, NY 10010-1710. Months of issue are March, June, September, and December. Periodicals postage paid at New York, NY, and additional mailing offices. Subscription price per year is $340.00 (US individuals), $582.00 (US institutions), $100.00 (US students), $371.00 (Canadian individuals), $669.00 (Canadian institutions), $100.00 (Canadian students), $470.00 (international individuals), $669.00 (international institutions), and $215.00 (international students). To receive student/resident rate, orders must be accompanied by name of affiliated institution, date of term, and the *signature* of program/residency coordinator on institution letterhead. Orders will be billed at individual rate until proof of status is received. Foreign air speed delivery is included in all *Clinics* subscription prices. All prices are subject to change without notice. **POSTMASTER:** Send address changes to *Foot and Ankle Clinics*, Elsevier Health Sciences Division, Subscription Customer Service, 3251 Riverport Lane, Maryland Heights, MO 63043. **Customer Service: 1-800-654-2452 (US and Canada). From outside of the United States and Canada, call 314-447-8871. Fax: 314-447-8029. E-mail: JournalsCustomerService-usa@ elsevier.com (for print support); JournalsOnlineSupport-usa@elsevier.com (for online support).**

Reprints. For copies of 100 or more, of articles in this publication, please contact the Commercial Reprints Department, Elsevier Inc., 360 Park Avenue South, New York, NY 10010-1710. Tel.: 212-633-3874; Fax: 212-633-3820; E-mail: reprints@elsevier.com.

Contributors

CONSULTING EDITOR

MARK S. MYERSON, MD
Executive Director and Founder, Steps2Walk, Baltimore, Maryland, USA

EDITOR

SUDHEER C. REDDY, MD
Orthopaedic Surgeon, Department of Orthopaedic Surgery, Shady Grove Orthopaedics, Adventist Medical Center, Adventist HealthCare, Medical Faculty Associates, George Washington University, Rockville, Maryland, USA

AUTHORS

AMIETHAB AIYER, MD
Chief of Foot and Ankle Surgery, Orthopaedic Surgery, University of Miami, Jackson Memorial Hospital, Miami, Florida, USA

DANIEL BAUMFELD, MD, PhD
Adjunct Professor, Federal University of Minas Gerais – UFMG, Foot and Ankle Surgeon, Felicio Rocho Hospital, Belo Horizonte, Minas Gerais, Brazil

JORGE BRICENO, MD
Foot and Ankle Service, Department of Orthopedic Surgery, Pontificia Universidad Catolica de Chile, Santiago, Chile

CESAR DE CESAR NETTO, MD, PhD
Assistant Professor, Department of Orthopedics and Rehabilitation, University of Iowa, Iowa City, Iowa, USA

JORGE JAVIER DEL VECCHIO, MD, MBA
Head, Foot and Ankle Section, Orthopaedics Department, Hospital Universitario - Fundación Favaloro, Department of Kinesiology and Physiatry, Universidad Favaloro, Ciudad Autónoma de Buenos Aires, Buenos Aires, Argentina; Minimally Invasive Foot and Ankle Society (GRECMIP-MIFAS), Merignac, France

JORGE FILIPPI, MD, MBA
Foot and Ankle Division, Department of Orthopedic Surgery, Clinica Las Condes, Santiago, Chile

MAURICIO ESTEBAN GHIOLDI, MD
Foot and Ankle Section, Orthopaedics Department, Hospital Universitario - Fundación Favaloro, Ciudad Autónoma de Buenos Aires, Argentina

WILLIAM A. HESTER III, MD
Foot and Ankle Fellow, Sidney Kimmel Medical College, Thomas Jefferson University, The Rothman Institute, Philadelphia, Pennsylvania, USA

GAVIN HEYES, FRCS, MSc
Consultant Trauma and Orthopaedic Surgeon, Trauma and Orthopaedics Department, Aintree University Hospital, Liverpool, United Kingdom

SHUYUAN LI, MD, PhD
Research and Program Coordinator, Steps2Walk, Baltimore, Maryland, USA

NACIME SALOMÃO BARBACHAN MANSUR, MD, PhD
Head of the Foot and Ankle Sector, Department of Orthopedics and Traumatology, Escola Paulista de Medicina, Sao Paulo Federal University, São Paulo, São Paulo, Brazil

PILAR MARTÍNEZ-DE-ALBORNOZ, MD
Orthopaedic Foot and Ankle Unit, Orthopaedic and Trauma Department, Hospital Universitario Quironsalud Madrid, Faculty of Medicine, UEM Madrid, Madrid, Spain

ANDY MOLLOY, FRCS, MD
Consultant Trauma and Orthopaedic Surgeon, Trauma and Orthopaedics Department, Aintree University Hospital, Liverpool, United Kingdom

MANUEL MONTEAGUDO, MD
Orthopaedic Foot and Ankle Unit, Orthopaedic and Trauma Department, Hospital Universitario QuironsaludMadrid, Faculty of Medicine, UEM Madrid, Madrid, Spain

MARK S. MYERSON, MD
Executive Director and Founder, Steps2Walk, Baltimore, Maryland, USA

CAIO AUGUSTO DE SOUZA NERY, MD, PhD
Foot and Ankle Sector Professor, Head of the Discipline of Orthopedics, Department of Orthopedics and Traumatology, Escola Paulista de Medicina, Sao Paulo Federal University, São Paulo, São Paulo, Brazil

DAVID I. PEDOWITZ, MS, MD
Associate Professor of Orthopaedic Surgery, Foot and Ankle Fellowship Director, Sidney Kimmel Medical College, Thomas Jefferson University, The Rothman Institute, Philadelphia, Pennsylvania, USA

TOMÁS ARAÚJO PRADO PEREIRA, MD
Foot and Ankle Department, Hospital Moinhos de Vento (HMV), Porto Alegre, Rio Grande do Sul, Brazil

SUDHEER C. REDDY, MD
Orthopaedic Surgeon, Department of Orthopaedic Surgery, Shady Grove Orthopaedics, Adventist Medical Center, Adventist HealthCare, Medical Faculty Associates, George Washington University, Rockville, Maryland, USA

MARTINUS RICHTER, MD, PhD
Professor, Department for Foot and Ankle Surgery Rummelsberg and Nuremberg, Location Hospital, Schwarzenbruck, Germany

JOSÉ ANTÔNIO VEIGA SANHUDO, MD, PhD
Coordinator, Head, Foot and Ankle Department, Hospital Moinhos de Vento (HMV), Porto Alegre, Rio Grande do Sul, Brazil

MAX SEITER, MD
Fellow, Sports Medicine Orthopaedic Surgery, Steadman Philippon Research Institute, Vail, Colorado, USA

EMILIO WAGNER, MD
Orthopedic Surgeon, Universidad de Desarrollo - Clinica Alemana de Santiago, Vitacura, Santiago, Chile

PABLO WAGNER, MD
Orthopedic Surgeon, Universidad de Desarrollo - Clinica Alemana de Santiago, Universidad de los Andes - Hospital Militar de Santiago, Vitacura, Santiago, Chile

ROBERTO ZAMBELLI, MD
Head of Orthopedic Department, Mater Dei Healthcare Network, Belo Horizonte, Minas Gerais, Brazil

Editorial Advisory Board

Contents

The interaction between hypermobility and hallux valgus remains both contemporary and incendiary. The difficulty in setting clinical and radiological parameters to diagnose and the complexity of questions that circumnutate the philosophy among etiology and denouement, fires up the debate regarding these conditions. Outcomes among procedures that address or neglect ray instability are still used as argument for any group of believers or nonbelievers. Through proving the true existence of hypermobility and its relationship with bunions, our colleges and professors have produced an incredible amount of excellent data that helped us better comprehend the hallux valgus syndrome in a general manner.

Health care costs are increasing. Funding is not increasing at a commensurate rate. Demonstrable cost-effectiveness is critical when selecting operation and implant type. Clinicians must justify their decision on surgery and implant type, providing patient-reported outcome measures (PROM). Providing such data on cost and PROM forms the basis of future cost-effectiveness analysis (CEA). Such analysis is complex. Future research should analyze cost variables individually. Day case surgery, multimodal analgesia, and simultaneous surgery for bilateral cases show promise in reducing cost. With evidence of increased recurrence, requirement for additional equipment and more expensive implants it is unlikely to demonstrate superior cost-effectiveness.

Hallux valgus (HV) represents a progressive 3-dimensional deformity that includes bone malalignment, hypermobility of the first ray, and imbalanced soft-tissue structures of the midfoot and forefoot. Conventional radiographs provide sectorized and limited information of the deformity in different planes. The literature evidence supporting the use of cone beam weightbearing computed tomography in the assessment of HV has been growing. It demonstrates important advances that include the ability to reliably perform traditional measurements such as HV angle and intermetatarsal angle in the 3-dimensional setting.

Anesthesia management during hallux valgus surgery trends toward multimodal pain control. Locoregional anesthesia with peripheral nerve blocks and wound instillation increase pain control. Peripheral nerve blocks as first-line analgesia are effective with minimal side effects. Local wound instillation has a variable but positive effect with minimal negative side effects. Nonsteroidal anti-inflammatory drugs in bone-to-bone healing remain controversial; however, they reduce opiate requirements and enhance patient satisfaction. Opiate agonists remain the mainstay for postoperative pain; long-acting formulations minimize pain crises. Multimodal analgesia with locoregional anesthesia facilitate the progress of hallux valgus surgery as an outpatient procedure.

Metatarsus adductus is common clinical entity with an estimated prevalence of approximately 30%. Multiple radiographic methods exist to evaluate the extent of the deformity, with the Sgarlato and Engel methods most commonly used. Surgical treatment varies, consisting of proximal versus distal metatarsal osteotomies, TMT arthrodesis, and realignment of the lesser rays. Particularly in severe cases, addressing all deformities is critical to obtaining a good outcome.

Coronal malalignment is an important deformity parameter in hallux valgus feet. Approximately 90% of patients with hallux valgus have some degree of metatarsal pronation. In operated hallux valgus, persistent metatarsal pronation is an independent deformity relapse factor. Coronal malalignment can be identified through an anteroposterior (AP) weight-bearing foot radiograph and a weight-bearing forefoot scan. The AP foot view can identify 3 levels of rotation: mild, moderate and severe metatarsal pronation. Regarding the treatment options, some techniques are capable of rotational correction, such as the proximal rotational metatarsal osteotomy, Lapidus, dome osteotomy, and proximal oblique sliding closing wedge.

Minimally invasive (MIS) or percutaneous surgery has evolved rapidly through the development of novel techniques with precise description, correct indications, and the incorporation of modifications of safe and effective techniques described in open surgery. The correct term to describe these procedures should be percutaneous and MIS should be reserved for procedures between percutaneous and open surgery (eg, osteosynthesis). According to results, third-generation techniques are useful, effective, and easier than open procedures. It seems that MIS surgery has an extensive learning curve, and therefore it may be difficult to duplicate the results shown on already-published data.

Hallux valgus is an extremely common and often disabling deformity. In addition to valgus deformity of the hallux, varying degrees of varus and supination of the first metatarsal and instability in the metatarsophalangeal and metatarsocuneiform joints are frequently present. Because of the complexity and multiplicity of deformities, surgical techniques and fixation methods continue to be developed to obtain better results. Recent studies have focused on correcting pronation of the first metatarsal as a way of correcting and equalizing the metatarsal sesamoid bones in a more horizontal and stable position, possibly minimizing the chance of recurrence of the deformity.

The evolution of Lapidus fixation has been strongly associated with the understanding of the anatomy and function of the first tarsometatarsal joint, the mechanism of hypermobility of the first tarsometatarsal joint, and cause of the hallux valgus deformity in 3 dimensions. Some methods, such as plantar plating, nitinol staples, and intramedullary fixation, have proven to be stronger biomechanically in cadaveric testing. Theoretically, stable fixation will reduce the rate of complications, in particular, that of nonunion and allow for early postoperative weight-bearing. Further clinical studies are needed to examine whether current biomechanical studies will translate to relevant clinical outcomes.

The hallux valgus is one of the most challenging foot and ankle deformities to correct. The current concept is to consider the hallux valgus as a triplane deformity, and the parameters in transverse, sagittal, and frontal planes must be considered. The hallux valgus angle, intermetatarsal angle, tibial sesamoid position, and lateral edge of the first metatarsal head are valuable parameters to evaluate to understand the magnitude of the deformity. Diaphyseal corrections, such as scarf, and proximal interventions, such as crescentic osteotomy and Lapidus arthrodesis, are the most powerful techniques to address triplane deformity, because they are able to correct all misalignments.

Postoperative management of hallux valgus varies widely. Setting preoperative expectations is an important aspect of attaining a successful outcome, but this is not routinely reviewed in the literature. This chapter offers suggestions on successfully navigating this area of patient care. Current concepts focus on pain control, immobilization, and return to activities. This chapter also reviews the current literature in these areas and sets out the authors' preferred management in the postoperative setting.

 Video content accompanies this article at http://www.foot.theclinics. com.

Complications following hallux valgus (HV) reconstruction will have an expected incidence of between 10% and 55% of cases. The more commonly reported complications include undercorrection/recurrence, overcorrection (hallux varus), transfer metatarsalgia, nonunion, malunion, avascular necrosis, arthritis, hardware removal, nerve injury, and ultimately patient dissatisfaction. The presence of arthritis will be an indication for fusion, whereas osteotomies will be the procedure of choice if the first metatarsophalangeal joint is healthy. Wide experience in primary HV surgery is advised before dealing with complex cases of failed HV surgery.

Avascular necrosis (AVN), nonunion, malunion, and metatarsophalangeal (MTP) osteoarthritis following hallux valgus osteotomies, as well as pathophysiology, diagnosis, prevention strategies, and treatment are discussed in this article. AVN and nonunion are very infrequent, and they can be effectively prevented taking into consideration local anatomy preservation, biomechanics, and patient comorbidities. Shortening, elevation, plantarflexion, varus/valgus, and rotational of the first metatarsal are the most common types of malunion. They can lead to pain, stiffness, deformity recurrence, and transfer metatarsalgia. MTP osteoarthritis can develop after metatarsal malunion or AVN. Treatment options include cheilectomy, osteotomies to correct malunions, and MTP arthrodesis.

FOOT AND ANKLE CLINICS

RELATED SERIES

Clinics in Sports Medicine
Orthopedic Clinics
Physical Medicine and Rehabilitation Clinics

Preface

Controversies in the Approach to Complex Hallux Valgus Correction

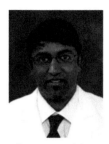

Sudheer C. Reddy, MD
Editor

Hallux valgus continues to remain a challenging condition to treat despite the myriad techniques available. Perhaps in no other disorder are the results as apparent to both the clinician and the patient. Successes and failures are apparent for both to see. Symptomatic hallux valgus can create frequent problems for the patient, including difficulty with shoe wear, walking, cosmetic concerns, and lesser toe pathologic conditions. Every aspect of management continues to be debated from the evaluation to the intraoperative and postoperative treatment.

The following issue is devoted to the recent advancements made in the field of hallux valgus. Topics include the use of weight-bearing imaging in the evaluation, current trends in anesthesia management, role of coronal plane malalignment, and the advent of minimally invasive surgery. Additional topics focus on the cost-effectiveness of surgical techniques, postoperative management, and complications, including hallux varus, metatarsophalangeal osteoarthritis, and malunion/nonunion. Newer topics, such as the evolution in the thinking of Lapidus fixation, and current trends in osteotomy fixation have been added.

I would like to sincerely thank the authors for their willingness and efforts in bringing this issue to fruition as well as to the staff at Elsevier for their assistance. A special thanks also goes to Mark Myerson not only for allowing me to be part of a wonderful project but also for his guidance and advice over the years as well as his enduring commitment to education, contributions to the field, and humanitarian outreach.

Foot Ankle Clin N Am 25 (2020) xv–xvi
https://doi.org/10.1016/j.fcl.2019.11.003
1083-7515/20/© 2019 Published by Elsevier Inc.

foot.theclinics.com

I hope that you enjoy this issue of *Foot and Ankle Clinics of North America* and that it can be of assistance in managing this complex condition.

Sudheer C. Reddy, MD
Shady Grove Orthopaedics
Adventist Health Care
Medical Faculty Associates
George Washington University
9601 Blackwell Road, Suite 100
Rockville, MD 20850, USA

E-mail address:
sreddy8759@yahoo.com

Hypermobility in Hallux Valgus

Nacime Salomão Barbachan Mansur, MD, PhD*,
Caio Augusto de Souza Nery, MD, PhD

KEYWORDS

- Hallux • Valgus • Hypermobility • Ray • Instability • Tarsometatarsal • Laxity
- Lapidus

KEY POINTS

- Decision over the best surgical procedure to treat severe and "abnormal" bunions has always been a matter of huge debate. The presence of a hypermobility as a contributive factor to the equation is still undetermined.
- There is still not enough data to determine first ray instability etiology and incidence. The higher rate of hypermobility in patients with hallux valgus lacks determination if the condition is cause or consequence.
- Several clinical and radiographic findings can help surgeons diagnose the instability presence and plan a proper treatment.
- Despite good articles supporting both the existence and the inexistence of first ray hypermobility, high evidence is still lacking and only represented by one clinical trial that did not endorsed the instability theory.
- The Lapidus fusion, modified or not, remains the surgeon's first choice when facing hypermobility. Although not absent of complications, this procedure has been demonstrating good and lasting results.

INTRODUCTION

Perhaps there is no subject as controversial as the association of hypermobility and hallux valgus (HV). Even its true existence is debatable, leading to more profound and unanswered questions, such as the genuine need for the condition direct surgical assessment and the real changes that this procedure produced in patient outcomes over the past years.

Does first ray hypermobility really exist? Does it need a fusion to be handled? Am I having better results by treating my patients with HV with a Lapidus procedure? These questions inhabit both fellows and senior surgeons' minds constantly and have no

Department of Orthopedics and Traumatology, Escola Paulista de Medicina, Sao Paulo Federal University, 715 Napoleao de Barros Street-1st Floor, Vila Clementino, São Paulo, São Paulo 04038002, Brazil
* Corresponding author.
E-mail address: nacime@nacime.com.br

Foot Ankle Clin N Am 25 (2020) 1–17
https://doi.org/10.1016/j.fcl.2019.10.004
1083-7515/20/© 2019 Elsevier Inc. All rights reserved.

definitive answer from the current literature. We humbly try to display the most complete disease scenario and possibly the next steps that are being taking in seeking those responses.

EPIDEMIOLOGY

Although a high HV prevalence has been shown in the literature, reaching approximately 20% to 35% of the adult population, the estimation of those who would sustain first ray hypermobility is not well defined.[1,2] Only a few studies can state that a higher degree of motion is present at the bunion population, without quantifying a percentage or ratio between groups.[3]

In a 2012 study by Biz and colleagues,[4] the investigators showed an up to 30% incidence in a population tested with the Klaue device. When a ballet dancer group was analyzed, a 45% of first ray hypermobility was found and a 81% sensitivity and specificity in relation to HV was reported.

Another article by Singh and colleagues[5] in 2016 found 81% of instability in patients with HV (with a 6.7 odds ratio) compared with a 24% occurrence in the control group. These results also were sustained by Klaue device measurements in 2 planes.

Even though we did not clearly identify how many patients have tarsometatarsal (TMT) instability, the Lapidus ratio of the procedures undertaken to treat the deformity was believed to be at a 10% proportion.[6–8] No new data picturing this procedure percentage in all HV surgeries has been published since then.

ETIOLOGY

First ray hypermobility etiology is often blurred by HV theories. Because we still do not comprehend the complete pathophysiology of this presentation, or either why only a percentage of patients with bunion are diagnosed with this instability, these perceptions can be flawed. Even theories that discuss if the hypermobility is the cause or consequence of HV are not yet clarified.

The literature understanding that intrinsic factor plays a much larger role in the HV development meets hypermobility necessity for explanation. As shoe wearing appears to only contribute to deformity worsening, the genetic predisposition (autosomal dominant inheritance with incomplete penetrance) gains more importance and may enlighten why patients could have different presentations when it comes to bunions.[8–10]

When speculating why ballet dancers and other athletes might have higher hypermobility rates, some investigators inferred that the stress related to activity and technique errors (pronation) may be responsible for this finding.[4,11]

The sole effect of the peroneus longus in the first ray axial and sagittal stability has received attention in the literature to demonstrate its importance over medial column pathogeneses.[12,13] Other studies claim attention to the misaligned peroneus longus, the plantar fascia, and other plantar ligamentous structures losing their biomechanical advantages, and, as a result, promoting an unstable first ray.[3,13]

General laxity (and its undoubtful genetic component) is another known reason for HV development as well for medial column hypermobility.[14–16] A mild ligament laxity might be present in up to 70% of woman with juvenile bunions and diseases that produces general severe ligamentous laxity as rheumatoid arthritis, Marfan, Ehler-Danos, and osteogenesis imperfecta also evolve with hypermobility and deformity.[10,17,18] Although this perception has been sustained by literature, no articles had the ability to show a true relation between these conditions and its possible results.[19]

The association between hypermobility and metatarsus primus varus returned to gain interest by investigators over the past years due the perception that TMT insta-bility occurs more in the axial (transverse) plane than in the sagittal level.[1,20,21] Again, there is still no information to conclude which is the protagonist and which is the corollary.

CLINICAL FINDINGS

Patients presenting hypermobility and HV will mostly seek a consultation due to bunion presence and the inherent predicaments that the deformity causes, as pain at the medial aspect of the hallux, local bursitis, and shoe wear difficulty.[9,22,23]

Besides the usual HV and possible associated conditions (such as lesser toe defor-mities), subjects with hypermobility may present subtle clinical findings (**Box 1**), most of them secondary to an unstable first ray.[11] Inspection can reveal a spoonlike hallux appearance (**Fig. 1**), caused by first metatarsal dorsal subluxation, and a lack of plantar keratosis under the first ray.[24–26] A second plantar hyperkeratosis might be portrayed, disclosing a lateral shift of the loading area.[27,28] Patients also must be examined for range of motion (ROM) in all joints in a search for generalized laxity, as well as for knee and hindfoot alignment because these structures have been related to the condition.[16]

During gait analysis, it is possible to observe a dynamic elevation of the first ray and a sag at the TMT joint. A pronation and an adduction by the first metatarsal at the late midstance phase may be perceived, especially when using tridimensional evalua-tions.[29] Palpation can produce pain under the second and third metatarsal heads, a consequence of the weight transfer. Discomfort at the TMT joint may be a sign of local-ized arthritis, a possible hypermobility late effect.[30]

The traditional direct maneuver to test ray mobility is by holding and stabilizing the intermediate and lateral columns of the foot with one hand (**Fig. 2**) while the other hand produces a dorsal-plantar translation with the medial column, as described by Morton. More than 10 mm in dislocation (or a complete dorsal overhaul) is considered positive.[31,32] This test, as the device created based on it, received a modification to reproduce the transverse instability. The ray is also shifted in a dorsal-medial direction.[4,33,34]

Pinching the first web space (using the index and the thumb) to provoke a free medial metatarsal displacement added to the ability to touch both fingers (**Fig. 3**) is

Box 1
Clinical Findings in Hipermobility
Hallux pronation
Dorsal first metatarsal migration
Spoonlike hallux
No first-ray plantar keratosis
Plantar-dorsal first translation greater than 10 mm
Pinch the first web space
Silfverskiöld test
Barouk test

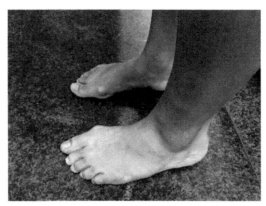

Fig. 1. Patient with HV and hypermobility showing a spoonlike hallux appearance caused by first metatarsal dorsal migration.

considered a sign of hypermobility. Strapping the forefoot and precipitating a deformity reduction in both clinical and radiological aspects is another indication of the condition.[30,35]

The presence of a tight Achilles tendon has been correlated with HV and hypermobility.[11,25,36] Therefore, its assessment remains important by properly checking the ankle ROM and searching for the contracture responsible with the *Silfverskiöld* test.[37] Barouk and colleagues[25,38] described a clinical maneuver to evaluate the presence of a dorsal first metatarsal migration and a failed windlass mechanism that could both generate HV and hallux rigidus.[24] The great toe limitation in dorsiflexion is naturally normalized by flexing the knee and relaxing the gastrocnemius muscle (**Fig. 4**).

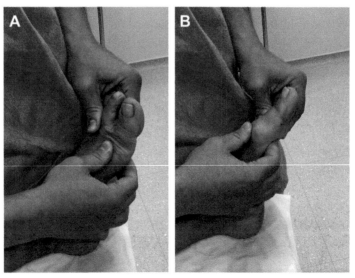

Fig. 2. Ray hypermobility tested by grasping the lateral and intermediate columns with one hand and producing a plantar (*A*) to dorsal (*B*) displacement. Note the ankle neutral position.

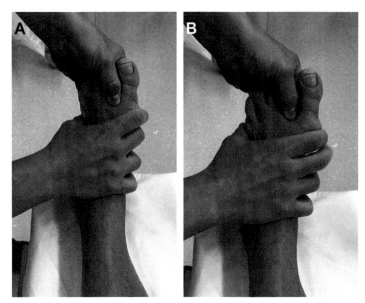

Fig. 3. First web space pinching test as described by Valderrabano and colleagues. The physician's thumb and index finger are placed between the first and second metatarsal heads (*A*). By pinching the space (*B*), it is possible to observe unrestrained first metatarsal medial displacement permitting the examiner's fingers to touch.

SUBSIDIARY EXAMS FINDINGS

Over the past years, researches tried to determine, reproduce, and quantify the first ray hypermobility perceived at clinical observations by using external devices (**Box 2**). Klaue and colleagues[39,40] were pioneers in attempting to achieve this goal. The investigators coined an 8-mm mark as a limit between a normal and a hypermobile ray. Glasoe and colleagues[31,41,42] later validated another apparatus intending to minimize their predecessors' problems by better stabilizing the foot and allowing the machine to translate the metatarsus.

Despite the difficulties in incorporating this device into clinical practice due their intrinsic high-cost, its incapacity in isolating the TMT joint and its problems in reproducing the proper axial instability, they were crucial in determining patterns and understanding the disease.[5,43–45]

Gait studies and multisegmented foot models have been seeking to identify differences between patients and diseases. From a simple pedobarography (**Fig. 5**) to a complex 3-dimensional computerized analysis, investigators observed patterns and possible instability signs.[21,28,29,46,47] Differences among genders concerning greater hallux pressure, faster timing, amid heel contact, first metatarsal load and a more medial pressure foot trajectory (lacking calcaneocuboid clutching and peroneus longus proper action) in girls were described as factors that might explain hypermobility.[28] Excessive rearfoot eversion and an altered intersegmental motion pattern between rearfoot and midfoot, by not locking the midtarsal joints, led to forefoot hypermobility during late stance.[29]

Radiographic signs are still being used by surgeons in an attempt to justify clinical observations through radiographic images. The frontal plane weight-bearing view may show an increase in the intercuneiform (IC) space, an oblique TMT joint, and second

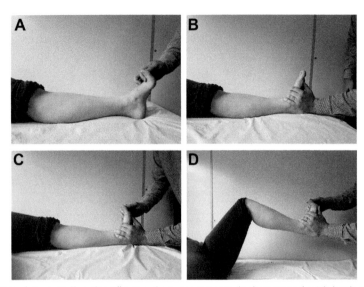

Fig. 4. Barouk test. Hallux dorsiflexion that seems normal when tested with both ankle and foot in plantar flexion (A) may exhibit limitation when assessed with the ankle in neutral (B, C). This is regularized when the knee is flexed and the gastrocnemius relaxes, allowing the big toe to move freely (D).

metatarsal cortical hypertrophy (**Fig. 6**). Lateral radiographs can demonstrate a first metatarsal dorsal migration and a gapping at the plantar aspect (**Fig. 7**) of the TMT joints (more than 2 mm). These incidences also should demonstrate joint arthritis, when present. Axial sesamoid view will display an important pronation in patients with hypermobility.[6,44,48–51]

However, some of the traditional signs described previously were discredit by the literature. Grebing and Coughlin[45] in 2004 demystified the correlation between hypermobility and second metatarsal cortical augmenting. Doty and Coughlin[52] questioned the TMT joint shape and its unreliable radiographic manifestations as predictors to

---

Box 2
Subsidiary Exams Findings in Hipermobility

Klaue/Glasoe devices measures over 8 mm

Lateral forefoot load

First plantar ray pressure diminished

Tarsometatarsal (TMT) arthritis

Oblique TMT joint?

Intercuneiform widening

Second metatarsal hypertrophy?

TMT plantar gapping

Dorsal first metatarsal migration

First metatarsal pronation, adduction and inversion

Left Mean Pressure   Right Mean Pressure

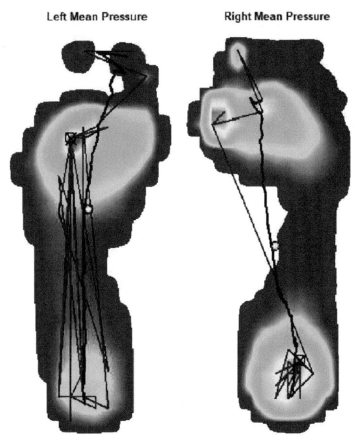

Fig. 5. Dynamic pedobarographic image in a patient with a left HV and a lateral normal aligned right hallux. Note the absence in first metatarsal load at the left side as well the weight transfer.

medial column instability. Glasoe and colleagues[53,54] also interrogated the first metatarsal dorsal translation as a sign of increased TMT mobility and their relations with foot conditions.[49]

As technology developed through the years, weight-bearing computed tomography (CT) **(Fig. 8)** has also been used in the study of first ray hypermobility.[1,12,20,44,50,55,56] Kimura and colleagues[1,20] showed an increase at the medial IC joint movement as well greater navicular dorsiflexion, superior medial cuneiform eversion, and a higher first metatarsal dorsiflexion, inversion, and adduction in patients with HV through their studies, arguing in favor of an instability in the entire first column.

Geng and colleagues[55] found a dorsiflexion, supination, and internal rotation of the metatarsal-cuneiform joint. The investigators claimed that hypermobility happens in multiple planes during HV deformity. Simons and colleagues contended the importance of the peroneus longus in maintaining medial longitudinal arch and claimed attention to the residual metatarsal rotation that may persist when the condition is not corrected via a TMT arthrodesis.[12]

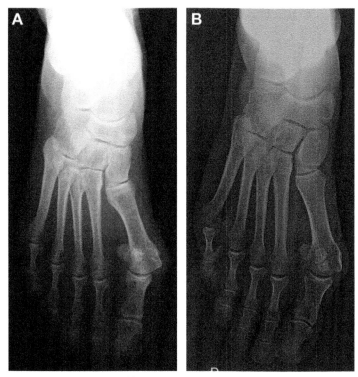

Fig. 6. Anteroposterior views in different patients exhibiting an oblique TMT joint configuration (A), opening of the IC space (B) and second metatarsal cortical hypertrophy (B).

CAUSE OR CONSEQUENCE?

One of the main efforts in research has been the debate over the hypermobility and its causality in relation to HV.[8,27,44,52,57–61] The major arguments for the consequence theorists are the incapacity to predict and determine the instability (by clinical or

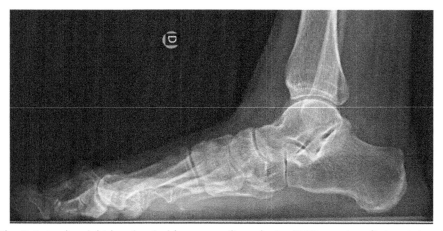

Fig. 7. Lateral weight-bearing incidence unveiling plantar TMT gapping, first metatarsal dorsal displacement and a hallux spoonlike.

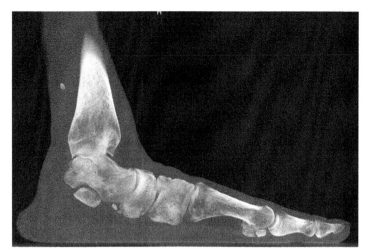

Fig. 8. Weight-bearing CT image clearly highlighting the first ray instability as the metatarsus pronates, adducts, and elevates. (*Courtesy of* Cesar de Cesar Netto, MD, PhD, Baltimore, MD and Weight-Bearing Computerized Tomography Group (WBCT).)

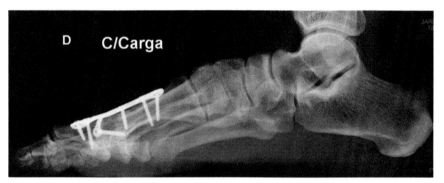

Fig. 9. MTP fusion showing correction in hypermobility radiographic patterns such as metatarsal dorsal migration and plantar gapping.

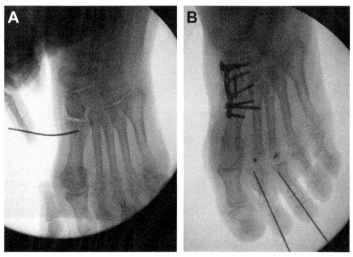

Fig. 10. Derotation capacity (*A*) of the Lapidus fusion as the metatarsal angle closes in, the sesamoids are reduced, and the head regains its angularity (*B*).

radiographic signs) and its natural and passive resolution after any osteotomy or meta-tarsophalangeal (MTP) fusion (**Fig. 9**). Hypermobility as origin was sustained by its be-lievers based in the tridimensional characteristic of the deformity (**Fig. 10**), the CORA concept (center of rotation of angulation), and the mystique over bunions that do not fit the usual presentation and outcomes.

Coughlin and colleagues[62,63] showed in cadaveric models and in patients treated by osteotomies combined with distal soft tissue procedures how the alleged mobility diminished after surgery, reaching normal values. They were followed by other inves-tigators who sustained the idea and also reported good correction results in addition to a low rate of complications and recurrence.[60] The plantar fascia stabilizing effect, restored by the previously described procedures, would normalize the ray instability and its possible deleterious effects.[64]

On the other hand, data were also produced raising questions about latent ray insta-bility.[6,8] Evolution in kinematic analysis by foot models and weight-bearing CT raised questions regarding hypermobility as an entity as stated before.[1,5,29] HV relation with

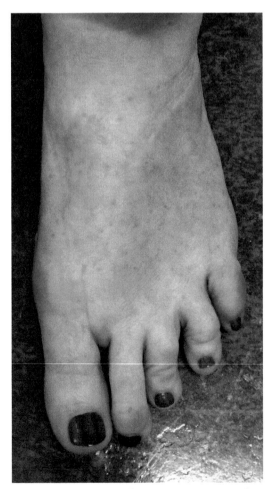

Fig. 11. Clinical foot appearance 5 years after an HV correction through a Lapidus TMT arthrodesis.

flatfoot, skew-foot, and other proximal deformities continues to emerge over literature and the concept of medial column stabilization remains decisive in fixing this scenario.[65–68]

OUTCOMES

Reasoning over hypermobility correction always has orbited the Lapidus TMT fusion. Since the first descriptions by Paul Lapidus, the ray stabilization through arthrodesis has been the answer to properly and reliably rectify deformity in all planes.[69,70] Several case series since then had shown consistent results, abiding corrections and a low complication rate.[26,61,71–74] The extremely small recurrence frequency over long follow-up periods (**Fig. 11**) has been the leading supporter's argument to defend the hypermobility existence.[27,71,75,76]

It is interesting to note the trends in surgeons choices coming from the original Lapidus (that included an arthrodesis between the first and second metatarsal bases), passing by the modified (**Fig. 12A**) procedure (only fusing the TMT1) and back to the classical author's concept (**Fig. 12B**) over the last decades. Studies improved the instability notion at the transverse plane, in other medial structures, and among intercuneiform joints provided ground for this technical change.[1,5,66,77] The search for stability and correction improvement as well as a faster recovery,

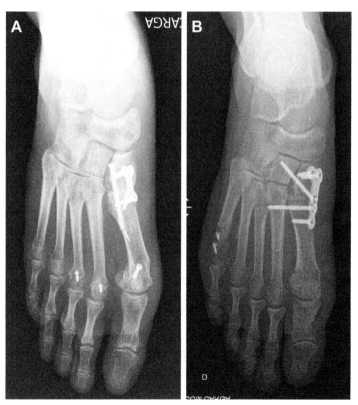

Fig. 12. Modified Lapidus fusion by only fixing and stabilizing the medial column (A). Original Lapidus arthrodesis (with modern implants) constructed by fusing the TMT1 and maintaining the medial to the intermediate column stabilized (B).

also resuscitated the column fixation idea.[30,78,79] Despite the hook test proposal of Fleming and colleagues,[77] this inclusion still remains a pure empiric decision, based mainly in radiographic indirect signs (IC opening and shape), intraoperative struggle in closing the intermetatarsal angle and abstract surgeon's feelings.

Although the TMT fusion thrived through the years, factors such as complications (**Fig. 13**), procedure morbidity, and specialist learning curve are until now an existing concern to both fellows and tutors. Albeit these matters are subestimated in the literature (as any poor surgical results that often suffer a publication bias), they are real and need to be contemplated when deciding the treatment.

Meanwhile, the only high-quality articles from which we can draw therapeutic conclusions remain the ones from Faber and colleagues[80,81] in 2004 and 2013. This

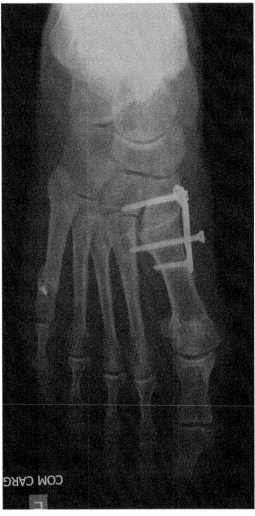

Fig. 13. Pseudoarthrosis, implant migration, and loss of correction after a TMT fusion using a medial plate. The patient received a modern anatomic implant and began an early weight-bearing protocol, as suggested by the current literature.

randomized clinical trial compared results and complications between the Hohmann osteotomy and the modified Lapidus fusion with 2 and 9 years of follow-up. A total of 101 feet (87 patients) were divided blindly into 2 groups and assessed by function and radiographic correction. The hypermobility presence and results were regressed analyzed and found to be similar in both sets. No difference was found in clinical and image outcomes among groups, even when ray instability presence was taken into consideration. This similarity continued for almost a decade and allowed investigators to advocate the nonexistence of the hypermobility theory.[80,81]

SUMMARY

Even after more than 20 years of good articles discrediting the hypermobility belief and its genuine relation with HV etiology and evolution, new data still emerge to confront this notion and the idea that instability is probably a disease consequence rather than an obscure cause.

When it comes to clinical evidence, facts still pends for the theory that claims mobility as an HV aftereffect. Hardly, we would say even impossibly, these will be the final and definitive words on the subject. Investigators continue to explore the hypermobility universe, attempting to minimize the inner voice that keeps saying "this is not an usual bunion."

DISCLOSURE

N.S.B. Mansur: nothing to disclose. C.A. de Souza Nery: consultant/speaker: Arthrex, Inc.

REFERENCES

1. Kimura T, Kubota M, Suzuki N, et al. Comparison of Intercuneiform 1-2 joint mobility between hallux valgus and normal feet using weightbearing computed tomography and 3-dimensional analysis. Foot Ankle Int 2018;39(3):355–60.
2. Nix S, Smith M, Vicenzino B. Prevalence of hallux abducto valgus in the general population: a systematic review. J Sci Med Sport 2010;12:e106.
3. Shibuya N, Roukis TS, Jupiter DC. Mobility of the first ray in patients with or without hallux valgus deformity: systematic review and meta-analysis. J Foot Ankle Surg 2017;56(5):1070–5.
4. Biz C, Favero L, Stecco C, et al. Hypermobility of the first ray in ballet dancer. Muscles Ligaments Tendons J 2012;2(4):282–8.
5. Singh D, Biz C, Corradin M, et al. Comparison of dorsal and dorsomedial displacement in evaluation of first ray hypermobility in feet with and without hallux valgus. Foot Ankle Surg 2016;22(2):120–4.
6. Schmid T, Krause F. The modified lapidus fusion. Foot Ankle Clin 2014;19(2): 223–33.
7. Sangeorzan BJ, Hansen ST. Modified lapidus procedure for hallux valgus. Foot Ankle 1989;9(6):262–6.
8. Smyth NA, Aiyer AA. Introduction: why are there so many different surgeries for hallux valgus? Foot Ankle Clin 2018;23(2):171–82.
9. Zirngibl B, Grifka J, Baier C, et al. Hallux valgus. Orthopade 2017;46(3):283–96.
10. Perera AM, Mason L, Stephens MM. The pathogenesis of hallux valgus. J Bone Joint Surg Am 2011;93(17):1650–61.
11. Davenport KL, Simmel L, Kadel N. Hallux valgus in dancers. J Dance Med Sci 2014;18(2):86–93.

12. Simons P, Dullaert K, Klos K, et al. The influence of the peroneus longus muscle on the foot under axial loading: a CT evaluated dynamic cadaveric model study. Clin Biomech 2016;34:7–11.
13. Rush SM, Christensen JC, Johnson CH. Biomechanics of the first ray. Part II: Metatarsus primus varus as a cause of hypermobility. A three-dimensional kinematic analysis in a cadaver model. J Foot Ankle Surg 2000;39(2):68–77.
14. Carl A, Ross S, Evanski P, et al. Hypermobility in hallux valgus. Foot Ankle Int 1988;8(5):264–70.
15. Al-Owain M, Al-Dosari MS, Sunker A, et al. Identification of a novel ZNF469 mutation in a large family with Ehlers-Danlos phenotype. Gene 2012;511(2):447–50.
16. Steinberg N, Finestone A, Noff M, et al. Relationship between lower extremity alignment and hallux valgus in women. Foot Ankle Int 2013;34(6):824–31.
17. Grahame R. Joint hypermobility and genetic collagen disorders: are they related? Arch Dis Child 1999;80(2):188–91.
18. Popelka S, Hromádka R, Vavík P, et al. Hypermobility of the first metatarsal bone in patients with Rheumatoid arthritis treated by lapidus procedure. BMC Musculoskelet Disord 2012;13. https://doi.org/10.1186/1471-2474-13-148.
19. Coughlin MJ. Hallux valgus. J Bone Joint Surg Am 1996;78(6):932–66.
20. Kimura T, Kubota M, Taguchi T, et al. Evaluation of first-ray mobility in patients with hallux valgus using weight-bearing CT and a 3-D analysis system a comparison with normal feet. J Bone Joint Surg Am 2017;99(3):247–55.
21. Dietze A, Bahlke U, Martin H, et al. First ray instability in hallux valgus deformity. Foot Ankle Int 2013;34(1):124–30.
22. Ferrari J. Hallux valgus (bunions). BMJ Clin Evid 2014;2014:1112.
23. Nery C, Coughlin MJ, Baumfeld D, et al. Hallux valgus in males–part 1: demographics, etiology, and comparative radiology. Foot Ankle Int 2013;34(5):629–35.
24. Maceira E, Monteagudo M. Functional hallux rigidus and the Achilles-calcaneus-plantar system. Foot Ankle Clin 2014;19(4):669–99.
25. Barouk LS. The effect of gastrocnemius tightness on the pathogenesis of juvenile hallux valgus: a preliminary study. Foot Ankle Clin 2014;19(4):807–22.
26. Fuhrmann RA. Die Korrekturarthrodese des ersten Tarsometatarsalgelenks zur Behandlung des fortgeschrittenen Spreizfußes mit Halluxvalgus-Fehlstellung. Oper Orthop Traumatol 2005;17(2):195–210.
27. Espinosa N, Wirth SH. Tarsometatarsal arthrodesis for management of unstable first ray and failed bunion surgery. Foot Ankle Clin 2011;16(1):21–34.
28. Ferrari J, Watkinson D. Foot pressure measurement differences between boys and girls with reference to hallux valgus deformity and hypermobility. Foot Ankle Int 2005;26:739–47.
29. Kawakami W, Takahashi M, Iwamoto Y, et al. Coordination among shank, rearfoot, midfoot, and forefoot kinematic movement during gait in individuals with hallux valgus. J Appl Biomech 2019;35(1):44–51.
30. Myerson MS. Reconstructive foot and ankle surgery. 2nd edition. Elsevier Saunders; 2010. https://doi.org/10.1016/C2009-0-32553-2.
31. Glasoe WM, Allen MK, Saltzman CL, et al. Comparison of two methods used to assess first-ray mobility. Foot Ankle Int 2002;23(3):248–52.
32. Voellmicke KV, Deland JT. Manual examination technique to assess dorsal instability of the first ray. Foot Ankle Int 2002;23:1040–1.
33. Glasoe WM, Yack HJ, Saltzman CL. Anatomy and biomechanics of the first ray. Phys Ther 1999;79(9):854–9.

34. Faber FW, Kleinrensink GJ, Verhoog MW, et al. Mobility of the first tarsometatarsal joint in relation to hallux valgus deformity: anatomical and biomechanical aspects. Foot Ankle Int 1999;20(10):651–6.
35. Romash MM, Fugate D, Yanklowit B. Passive motion of the first metatarsal cuneiform joint: Preoperative assessment. Foot Ankle 1990;10(6):293–8.
36. Dalmau-Pastor M, Yasui Y, Calder JD, et al. Anatomy of the inferior extensor retinaculum and its role in lateral ankle ligament reconstruction: a pictorial essay. Knee Surg Sports Traumatol Arthrosc 2016;24(4):957–62.
37. Silfverskiold N. Reduction of the uncrossed two-joints muscles of the leg to one-joint muscles in spastic conditions. Acta Chir Scand 1923;56:315–30.
38. Barouk LS, Barouk P. Hallux valgus et Gastrocnemiens courts: étude de deux series cliniques. In: Briéveté Des Gastrocnémiens. Montpellier (France): Sauramps Medical; 2012. p. 265–8.
39. Klaue K. Hallux valgus and hypermobility of the first ray–causal treatment using tarso-metatarsal reorientation arthrodesis. Ther Umsch 1991;48(12):817–23 [in German].
40. Klaue K, Hansen ST, Masquelet AC. Clinical, quantitative assessment of first tarsometatarsal mobility in the sagittal plane and its relation to hallux valgus deformity. Foot Ankle Int 1994;15(1):9–13.
41. Glasoe WM, Yack HJ, Saltzman CL. Measuring first ray mobility with a new device. Arch Phys Med Rehabil 1999;80(1):122–4.
42. Glasoe WM, Grebing BR, Beck S, et al. A comparison of device measures of dorsal first ray mobility. Foot Ankle Int 2005;26:957–61.
43. Grebing BR, Coughlin MJ. The effect of ankle position on the exam for first ray mobility. Foot Ankle Int 2004;25:467–75.
44. Doty JF, Harris WT. Hallux valgus deformity and treatment: a three-dimensional approach. Foot Ankle Clin 2018;23(2):271–80.
45. Grebing BR, Coughlin MJ. Evaluation of Morton's theory of second metatarsal hypertrophy. J Bone Joint Surg Am 2004;86-A(7):1375–86.
46. Wong DWC, Zhang M, Yu J, et al. Biomechanics of first ray hypermobility: an investigation on joint force during walking using finite element analysis. Med Eng Phys 2014;36(11):1388–93.
47. Kernozek TW, Elfessi A, Sterriker S. Clinical and biomechanical risk factors of patients diagnosed with hallux valgus. J Am Podiatr Med Assoc 2003;93(2):97–103.
48. Coughlin MJ, Saltzman CL, Nunley JA. Angular measurements in the evaluation of hallux valgus deformities : a report of the Ad Hoc Committee of the American Orthopedic Foot & Ankle Society on Angular Measurements. Foot Ankle Int 2002; 23(1):68–74.
49. Doty JF, Coughlin MJ, Hirose C, et al. First metatarsocuneiform joint mobility: radiographic, anatomic, and clinical characteristics of the articular surface. Foot Ankle Int 2014;35(5):504–11.
50. Welck MJ, Al-Khudairi N. Imaging of hallux valgus. Foot Ankle Clin 2018;23(2): 183–92.
51. King DM, Toolan BC. Associated deformities and hypermobility in hallux valgus : an investigation with weightbearing radiographs. Foot Ankle Int 2004;25:251–5.
52. Doty JF, Coughlin MJ. Hallux valgus and hypermobility of the first ray: facts and fiction. Int Orthop 2013;37(9):1655–60.
53. Glasoe WM, Allen MK, Saltzman CL. First ray dorsal mobility in relation to hallux valgus deformity and first intermetatarsal angle. Foot Ankle Int 2001;22(2): 98–101.

54. Glasoe WM, Allen MK, Kepros T, et al. Dorsal first ray mobility in women athletes with a history of stress fracture of the second or third metatarsal. J Orthop Sports Phys Ther 2002;32(11):560–7.
55. Geng X, Wang C, Ma X, et al. Mobility of the first metatarsal-cuneiform joint in patients with and without hallux valgus: in vivo three-dimensional analysis using computerized tomography scan. J Orthop Surg Res 2015;10(1):1–7.
56. Campbell B, Miller MC, Williams L, et al. Pilot study of a 3-dimensional method for analysis of pronation of the first metatarsal of hallux valgus patients. Foot Ankle Int 2018;39(12):1449–56.
57. Oravakangas R, Leppilahti J, Laine V, et al. Proximal opening wedge osteotomy provides satisfactory midterm results with a low complication rate. J Foot Ankle Surg 2016;55(3):456–60.
58. Dayton P, Kauwe M, Feilmeier M. Is our current paradigm for evaluation and management of the bunion deformity flawed? A discussion of procedure philosophy relative to anatomy. J Foot Ankle Surg 2015;54(1):102–11.
59. Smith BW, Coughlin MJ. The first metatarsocuneiform joint, hypermobility, and hallux valgus: what does it all mean? Foot Ankle Surg 2008;14(3):138–41.
60. Kim J, Park JS, Hwang SK, et al. Mobility changes of the first ray after hallux valgus surgery: clinical results after proximal metatarsal chevron osteotomy and distal soft tissue procedure. Foot Ankle Int 2008;29:468–72.
61. Kopp FJ, Patel MM, Levine DS, et al. The modified lapidus procedure for hallux valgus: a clinical and radiographic analysis. Foot Ankle Int 2005;26(11):913–7.
62. Coughlin MJ, Jones CP, Viladot R, et al. Hallux valgus and first ray mobility: a cadaveric study. Foot Ankle Int 2004;25(8):537–44.
63. Coughlin M, Jones CP. Hallux valgus and first ray mobility. J Bone Joint Surg Am 2007;1887–98. https://doi.org/10.2106/JBJS.F.01139.
64. Van Beek C, Greisberg J. Mobility of the first ray: review article. Foot Ankle Int 2012;32(9):917–22.
65. Hagmann S, Dreher T, Wenz W. Skewfoot. Foot Ankle Clin 2009;14(3):409–34.
66. Blackwood S, Gossett L. Hallux valgus/medial column instability and their relationship with posterior tibial tendon dysfunction. Foot Ankle Clin 2018;23(2):297–313.
67. Aiyer AA, Shariff R, Ying L, et al. Prevalence of metatarsus adductus in patients undergoing hallux valgus surgery. Foot Ankle Int 2014;35(12):1292–7.
68. Loh B, Chen JY, Yew AKS, et al. Prevalence of metatarsus adductus in symptomatic hallux valgus and its influence on functional outcome. Foot Ankle Int 2015;36(11):1316–21.
69. Lapidus PW. A quarter of a century of experience with the operative correction of the metatarsus varus primus in hallux valgus. Bull Hosp Joint Dis 1956;17(2):404–21.
70. Lapidus PW. The author's bunion operation from 1931 to 1959. Clin Orthop 1960;16:119–35.
71. Rink-Brüne O. Lapidus arthrodesis for management of hallux valgus - a retrospective review of 106 cases. J Foot Ankle Surg 2004;43(5):290–5.
72. Myerson MS, Badekas A. Hypermobility of the first ray. Foot Ankle Clin 2000;5(3):469–84.
73. Michels F, Guillo S, de Lavigne C, et al. The arthroscopic Lapidus procedure. Foot Ankle Surg 2011;17(1):25–8.
74. Bierman RA, Christensen JC, Johnson CH. Biomechanics of the first ray. Part III. Consequences of Lapidus arthrodesis on peroneus longus function: a three-

dimensional kinematic analysis in a cadaver model. J Foot Ankle Surg 2001; 40(3):125–31.

75. Klos K, Wilde CH, Lange A, et al. Modified Lapidus arthrodesis with plantar plate and compression screw for treatment of hallux valgus with hypermobility of the first ray: a preliminary report. Foot Ankle Surg 2013;19(4):239–44.

76. Gutteck N, Savov P, Panian M, et al. Preliminary results of a plantar plate for Lapidus arthrodesis. Foot Ankle Surg 2018;24(5):383–8.

77. Fleming JJ, Kwaadu KY, Brinkley JC, et al. Intraoperative evaluation of medial intercuneiform instability after lapidus arthrodesis: intercuneiform hook test. J Foot Ankle Surg 2015;54(3):464–72.

78. Galli MM, McAlister JE, Berlet GC, et al. Enhanced lapidus arthrodesis: crossed screw technique with middle cuneiform fixation further reduces sagittal mobility. J Foot Ankle Surg 2015;54(3):437–40.

79. Young NJ, Zelen CM. New techniques and alternative fixation for the Lapidus arthrodesis. Clin Podiatr Med Surg 2013;30(3):423–34.

80. Faber FWM, Mulder PGH, Verhaar JAN. Role of first ray hypermobility in the outcome of the Hohmann and the Lapidus procedure. A prospective, randomized trial involving one hundred and one feet. J Bone Joint Surg Am 2004;86-A(3): 486–95.

81. Faber FWM, van Kampen PM, Bloembergen MW. Long-term results of the Hohmann and Lapidus procedure for the correction of hallux valgus. Bone Joint J 2013;95-B(9):1222–6.

Cost-Effectiveness of Surgical Techniques in Hallux Valgus

Andy Molloy, FRCS, MD*, Gavin Heyes, FRCS, Msc

KEYWORDS

- Cost-effectiveness • Bunion • Hallux valgus surgery

KEY POINTS

- Health care costs are on the increase; however, funding is not increasing at a commensurate rate. Therefore demonstrable cost-effectiveness is critical when selecting operation and implant type.
- Cost-effectiveness analysis (CEA) in hallux valgus surgery is severely lacking in the literature. Such analysis is complex to set up, involving multiple cost variables.
- pragmatic approach to CEA research should involve looking at cost variables individually. Therefore, day case surgery, multimodal analgesia, and simultaneous surgery for bilateral cases show promise in safely reducing cost.
- There is no CEA for minimally invasive surgery for hallux valgus. With some evidence of increased recurrence, requirement for additional equipment and more expensive implants it is unlikely to demonstrate superior cost-effectiveness.

HEALTH CARE COSTS

In these times of austerity there has never been a greater need to deliver efficient and effective health care.

Health care costs are on the increase. In the United States, health care costs consumed around 4% of annual income in 1960. This cost increased by 0.5% to 6% in 2013, and in 2017 health care costs as a function of gross domestic product were thought to be in the region of 17.9%. Part of this is because of a reliance on private health insurance, high hospital fees, and running costs. Administration costs have also greatly increased and this is thought to be as a result of the complexity of billing.[1]

Regarding health care costs in Europe, they are organized and financed in differing ways. Germany, France, and Sweden have the highest percentage expenditure at 11% to 11.2%. The United Kingdom spends 9.8% of its gross domestic product on

Trauma and Orthopaedics Department, Aintree University Hospital, Lower Lane, Liverpool L9 7AL, UK
* Corresponding author.
E-mail address: andy.molloy@aintree.nhs.uk

Foot Ankle Clin N Am 25 (2020) 19–29
https://doi.org/10.1016/j.fcl.2019.10.005   foot.theclinics.com
1083-7515/20/© 2019 Elsevier Inc. All rights reserved.

health care.[2] However, the cost per person differs significantly, with France spending 3600 euros, Germany and Sweden over 4000 euros, and Switzerland spending most per person at over 5000 euros.[3] Secondary to demographic development, projected costs in Europe are set to increase between 0.7% and 3.8% of gross domestic product from 2007 to 2060.[4]

Regardless of the type of health care system in place and source of funding, costs are on a sustained and progressive increase. Therefore, not only is it crucial to make best use of limited resources, but also to return patients to the workforce as promptly and safely as possible. To do this, all treatment modalities should be continually assessed for their efficacy, durability, and performance, while also being compared with the established gold standard.

EVALUATING HALLUX VALGUS COST-EFFECTIVENESS

Surgery to correct hallux valgus is a commonly performed procedure; however, despite this there is a relative paucity of evidence in the literature supporting its cost-effectiveness.[5] One of the reasons for this is that defining the prevalence of hallux valgus is challenging. Hallux valgus pooled estimates for prevalence is 23%, but reports of prevalence range from 21% to 70%.[6–9]

Diagnostic criteria for hallux valgus in the literature are variable and populations are not all matched for age, sex, and foot wear type and use. This makes it difficult to define the total disease and financial burden for health services. There is a clear preponderance of hallux valgus in women.[6] Its prevalence also increases with age.[6] With the aging (65–84 years) population forecast to increase by 50% in the next 12 years,[10] the prevalence of hallux valgus is likely to increase at a commensurate rate. Although it is not generally a condition that leads to time off work owing to pain or inability to walk, significant deformity has been shown to increase the risk of falling in the elderly.[11]

Because of the lack of strong evidence of cost-effectiveness for hallux valgus surgery and the increased focus on getting the "greatest bang for your buck," many trusts in the United Kingdom have placed restrictions on providing hallux valgus surgery. Their policies stipulate that surgery should only be performed for progressive pain, deformity, and significant functional impairment despite optimal conservative management for at least 6 months and/or significant involvement of the second toe, neuritis, ulceration, or inflammatory process.[12–15]

In the United States, 1 study on the economic burden of foot and ankle operations in Medicare patients found that cost increased by 38% over the past 10 years. Furthermore, most of that cost was due to time out of work. This is a difficult factor to assess globally as health care systems, sick leave, and government allowances differ vastly.

Following recent changes due to the Affordable Care Act, reimbursement stratification has changed, with many treatments falling under the umbrella of routine foot care becoming exempt. For most, treatment of hallux valgus does not fall into this category; however, there is considerable geographic variation.

Therefore, to continue to justify current elective practices in Orthopedics, and in particular hallux valgus surgery, we must all demonstrate the ability to provide cost-effectiveness analysis (CEA) to our employers.

AVAILABLE METHODS OF COST-EFFECTIVENESS ANALYSIS

Deciding on the appropriate method(s) for assessment of cost-effectiveness is a challenge. Cost-effectiveness of surgical interventions requires assessment of more variables than just surgical intervention. For example, surgical interventions incur a high cost for a short period of time during the entirety of a patient's treatment. Other points to consider are the cost of postoperative rehabilitation, increased outpatient reviews (with imaging), additional operations, and the relative immediacy of surgical interventions to improve symptoms.

In the United States the Center for Evaluation of Value and Risk in health has set up a CEA registry. Their mission statement is "To inform the national debate on clinical and public health policy issues and to directly influence the prioritization of healthcare resources both domestically and globally."[16] However, there is not enough evidence in the literature on cost-effectiveness of hallux valgus surgery to feature in the CEA. With increasing demand to justify decision making, implant choice, and to provide demonstrable outcomes, registries like this will maintain high standards in data collection and will be vital to guide and defend surgical treatment.

In 2016, a panel of experts on cost-effectiveness in health and medicine (CEHM) gathered for a second time to redevelop a set of recommendations on how to assess cost-effectiveness by consensus opinion. The panel recommended the following:[17]

- All studies should report reference case series. In the reference series, parameters should be identified and definitions for cost-effectiveness provided.
  - For the purposes of this paper we decided to perform a CEA on a sample of our own patients. Patient-reported outcome measure (PROM) scores were collected in patients treated by either Scarf osteotomy, 1st metatarsalphalangeal joint (MTPJ) fusion, and Lapidus fusion. Costs for implants were collected from the National Health Service health care systems, as were estimated costs for day case and single-night length of stay.
- Following data collection, a summary of analysis in a conventional format as an incremental cost-effectiveness ratio should be formulated. Alternatively, net monetary benefit or net health benefit should be reported. Reimbursements to the health care provider should be reported.
- There should be an inclusion of an inventory of societal or nonhealth-related costs, such as cost incurred by patient (transport cost, carer cost, employment, and pay issues). If possible they should be quantified.
- There should be reporting of reference cases and these should include other perspectives and their respective differences, such as source of funding (public or private). In addition, there must be transparency with such differences.
- In terms of actual cost-effectiveness measurement, CEA should be measured in terms of quality-adjusted life years (QALYs). Quality measurements should be clearly weighted and scaled.
- Any CEA should incorporate additional costs to patient or health care provider, whether at the time of treatment or on subsequent follow-up.[17]

However, there are some issues with the use of QALYs as part of a cost-effectiveness measure. Depending on the source of funding, some organizations do not recognize the use of QALYs. In the United States, Medicare is not allowed to consider cost-effectiveness as part of their decision making process regarding funding of new diagnostic tests or surgical procedures. In addition, the Affordable Care Act also prohibited the use of a cost per QALY ratio as a threshold for cost-effectiveness and subsequent funding.[17–19]

On review of the literature, orthopedic papers studying cost-effectiveness have done so in differing ways. One paper evaluated cost-effectiveness of alternate hip bearings in total hip replacement. They looked at the cost for surgery outpatient follow-up and any revisions performed. The endpoint was death either owing to total hip replacement-related problems or death unrelated to the total hip replacement.[20]

They used the recommendations set out by the first CEHM panel meeting.[21] QALYs were used as a health utility assessment. Utility values for what qualified as a successful total hip arthroplasty were drawn from utility values already published in the literature. Although a hip arthroplasty paper, their results are applicable in CEA in other areas of orthopedics. They highlight the specific difficulty of evaluating implant choice and cost-effectiveness, in particular the time-consuming nature of follow-up until failure in such analysis.

Other papers have evaluated cost-effectiveness in comparison with nonoperative or suboptimal treatments. In addition, the time frame of studies and their endpoints are extremely variable.[22,23] Most CEA in the orthopedic literature is on hip and or knee arthroplasty. There is an underreporting of foot and ankle surgery cost-effectiveness.[22] The unifying feature of most good-quality hip and knee arthroplasty cost-effectiveness research is the use of recommendations set out by CEHM. In addition, they reported considerable variation in cost-effectiveness for revision surgery and "additional costs," such as antibiotic prophylaxis and blood product use. This is of interest to those informed in foot and ankle CEA as it highlights the importance of standardization of treatments where possible. Otherwise other cost variables (like antibiotic choice) could complicate primary cost variables, such as implant choice, and lead to the construction of complicated and large studies to suitably evaluate cost-effectiveness.

One systematic review has been published that assesses cost-effectiveness in general foot and ankle surgery. The study restricted their review to US papers on the standardization of costs and legislature that may dictate surgical treatment. Four studies were identified, 3 comparing total ankle replacement (TAR) with arthrodesis and or nonoperative treatment and 1 comparing screw and button fixation. All reported cost per QALY and although they reported significant differences in cost-effectiveness there was debate as to what constitutes an appropriate cost difference threshold.[23] Neither the review nor the individual papers commented in sufficient detail on whether or not return to work was significantly different between cohorts. In addition, return to work/loss of pay was not factored into their cost-effectiveness analyses. Further issues contributing to complexity in CEA was highlighted by a recent expert opinion seminar.[24] This raised the important question of when should we draw the line with study endpoints in CEA. They used the example of ankle arthrodesis versus TAR and asked whether progression of adjacent joint degeneration and implant failure through normal wear, both leading to further surgery, should be taken into consideration.

Regarding current cost-effectiveness research in hallux valgus surgery, there have been few papers published. In fact, cost-effectiveness studies of any kind centered on the hallux valgus are few and far between. One study used a cost-effectiveness ratio; a ratio of cost (dollars) over difference in clinical outcomes using the American Orthopaedic Foot and Ankle Society (AOFAS) score.[1] They compared Chevron, modified Scarf, Ludloff, proximal oblique sliding closing wedge osteotomies, and Lapidus fusion. They evaluated costs, including implants, hospital charges, radiographic charges, and medication use. They had incomplete data regarding complication and reoperation costs, but estimated these costs and calculated a global average. Their assigned complication reoperation rate was 5 (2.5%) in mild to moderate hallux valgus and 10 (5%) in severe hallux valgus. Clinic and hospital fees were averaged across all participating sites. Differences in AOFAS scores were calculated from preoperative scores and final score before discharge. Overall Chevron and modified Scarf osteotomies were most effective. This study is the first to report cost-effectiveness in surgery for hallux valgus. Although the reliability and sensitivity of the use of AOFAS score in hallux valgus has been questioned,[25,26] this study still provides important data regarding cost-effectiveness.

One further study in the cost-effectiveness of hallux valgus has been published.[27] This prospective study looked at 95 patients and evaluated cost-effectiveness by calculating a QALY. They used the Euroqol 5D (EQ5D) PROM score, took the difference preoperatively and postoperatively and then estimated a 15- and 20-year cumulative QALY improvement. This total was divided by an average cost for hallux valgus surgery, there was no reference to different fixation methods or additional procedures. This study reported cost-effectiveness on a par with hip and knee surgery; however, many assumptions have been made regarding the sustainability of a fairly constant PROM score over years (discounted rate of only 3.5% was assumed) and the absence of further procedures.

In addition to differences in cost-effectiveness based on method of treatment and fixation of the hallux valgus, one must also consider other methods of reducing cost, such as bilateral surgery and outpatient surgery. For over 20 years there have been publications favoring bilateral surgery. Early papers were small retrospective studies, they reported no difference in correction, complication rate, or patient satisfaction when compared with staged unilateral procedures. Therefore, it was suggested that there was no increased risk to the patient and improved cost-effectiveness to both the patient and health care provider.[28–30]

More recently, larger prospective studies have further substantiated this finding.[31,32] One UK-based study reported equivocal Manchester Oxford Foot Questionnaire (MOXFQ) scores and SF 36 scores between unilateral and bilateral surgery at 8-year follow-up using a questionnaire. There was no significant difference in complication rate between unilateral and bilateral cases; however, there was no CEA.[32]

Fridman and colleagues[33] also performed a comparative study of unilateral versus bilateral hallux valgus surgery. Not only did they find no difference in early complication rate, activity of daily living, and the visual analog score (VAS) for pain or patient satisfaction, they also formally assessed cost-effectiveness. They calculated average cost for surgeon, anesthesiologist, and hospital stay. In US dollars, single unilateral cases cost $3100, staged cases $6200, and simultaneous bilateral cases $4525. That is a cost saving of just under 26%.

Hallux valgus surgery is now commonly performed as a day case (outpatient or ambulatory) and there is evidence to support this. From a cost-effectiveness stand point, 1 large retrospective Spanish study used a weighted care unit to evaluate cost. They evaluated 292 day cases and 461 overnight stays. Both groups were comparable regarding diagnosis, severity, and intervention, and the day case procedure maintained a high patient satisfaction rating of 84.6 out of 100. A significant difference between weighted care unit spending was found, with increased spending in the overnight stay group.[34]

In 1 large randomized controlled study of 211 patients by Torkki and colleagues,[35,36] independent of the type of surgical intervention performed, when compared with orthotic treatment and control, at 2 years the cost for the surgery group was $1121.70; $1104.60 for the orthotic group and $1281.0 for the control group. Interestingly, there were significantly more visits to the physician in the control group. There was no difference in foot pain or footwear problems between groups; however, cosmetic appearance and patient satisfaction were significantly greater in the surgical group.

Day case surgery is now reported routinely in the literature and uniformly seems to have good patient-reported outcomes.[37] Factors that could influence length of stay in hospital should be considered when attempting to optimize cost-effectiveness. Such factors may include simultaneous bilateral surgery and specialist anesthetic techniques that lead to an increased number of day case procedures.

Although CEA was not performed, 1 study demonstrated that day case surgery in bilateral cases can deliver high PROM scores on a par with unilateral surgery and, more importantly, they demonstrated that bilateral surgery can be performed safely.[38] This is important because, intuitively, one would expect simultaneous surgery to be cheaper and less resource intensive than staged bilateral surgery.

To maximize the rate of successful day surgery discharge, patient analgesia needs to be optimized. Perioperative local analgesia can significantly influence postoperative pain. One randomized study compared combination local analgesia in the form of ropivacaine, morphine, ketorolac, and epinephrine compared with normal saline and demonstrated significantly improved analgesia that was sustained to 1 to 2 days postoperatively.[39] Following hallux valgus surgery, optimal oral analgesia is critical in reducing length of stay, readmission rate, and optimizing cost-effectiveness. Brattwal and colleagues[40] performed a randomized control trial comparing tramadol and etoricoxib in 98 patients and found greater pain relief with etoricoxib. All patients were discharged 2 hours postoperatively and there were no readmissions. Pricing for each medication differed depending on country, but was generally similar: approximately $1 per tablet.

Minimally Invasive Surgery

Proponents of minimally invasive surgery report that it is a valid procedure, particularly for bilateral surgery.[41] However, 1 systematic review reported recurrence as the most common complication, with a higher rate of occurrence when compared with conventional osteotomy methods.[42] Once again these outcomes, along with training and access to specialist equipment, will diminish the cost-effectiveness of minimally invasive procedures. At present, there is no CEA published in the literature regarding minimally invasive hallux valgus surgery. In addition there is a large degree of heterogenicity between studies regarding standardization of procedure, inclusion of additional forefoot procedures, analgesia, patient-reported outcomes, reporting of complications, and length of follow-up.[41–44] Consequently, national guidelines in the United Kingdom state that minimally invasive surgery should only be performed as part of a national study or audit, because efficacy and cost-effectiveness have not yet been definitely proven.[13,14]

Given the relative paucity of cost-effectiveness data in the literature we reviewed a sample of our own patients to ascertain a better idea of cost differences for Scarf osteotomies, 1st MTPJ fusions, and Lapidus fusions. We used the most straightforward and reproducible method of cost-effectiveness evaluation currently published. We calculated the cost (in dollars) for each single point PROM score improvement, as described previously by Wagner and colleagues.[1]

We used a sample of our own patients followed-up for at least 1 year, with prospective PROMs data. We collected PROMS from 56 patients (20 Scarf, 20 MTPJ fusions, and 16 Lapidus fusions). The PROMs collected were MOXFQ, the EQ5D, and VAS for pain.

Table 1 lists the mean cost of implants for each procedure, the cost for a day case stay in hospital and the cost for an overnight stay in hospital. Hospital stay cost estimates include theater, anesthetic, nursing, ward bed, and physiotherapy costs. We have not included any plastering, postoperative footwear, or outpatient costs. Costs are listed in dollars. Current market exchange rate at the time of writing paper was 1 US Dollar (0.765 British pound sterling).

Table 1
Costings for surgery (dollars)

Healthcare System	Mean Scarf Screw Cost (Range)	Mean 1st MTPJ Fusion Plate and Screws Cost (Range)	Mean Lapidus Plate and Screws Cost (Range)	Cost of Day Case Hospital Stay	Cost of an Overnight Stay in Hospital
United Kingdom (National Health Service)	102.5 (87.6–117.6)	755 (600–910)	830 (680–980)	888.9	1490

Table 2
Estimated total costs

Procedure	Total Cost of Day Surgery	Total Cost of Overnight Stay	Overall Mean Total Cost
Scarf	1093.9	1695	1093.9
1st MTPJ fusion	1643.9	2245	1643.9
Lapidus procedure	1718.9	2320	1831.6

Table 2 demonstrates the total costs for surgery (using mean prices) as a day case and surgery as an overnight stay. For the Scarf procedure we are working off a cost for 2 screws. In our sample of 56 patients, none of those receiving Scarf or 1st MTPJ fusions stayed overnight, therefore overall mean total cost is as stated in the total cost of day surgery. Three of the 16 patients receiving Lapidus required an overnight stay for mobility issues, hence the overall mean total cost of $1831.60.

Table 3 demonstrates the mean differences (highlighted in bold) in preoperative and postoperative PROM scores from our sample of 56 patients. The table also includes the cost in dollars per 1-point improvement in proms score. EQ5D scores work on a scale between 0 and 1; therefore, a 0.01 improvement is considered a 1-point improvement for the purposes of this study. Note that our EQ5D went up after Scarf

Table 3
Mean Patient-reported outcome measure score pre and post surgery

PROM Score	Scarf Score	Scarf Cost/Point	1st MTPJ Fusion	1st MTPJ Fusion Cost/Point	Lapidus	Lapidus Cost/Point
Preoperative MOXFQ pain	54.7		53.8		57.1	
Postoperative MOXFQ pain	28.8		28.3		47.3	
Difference in MOXFQ pain	25.9	42.24	25.5	64.67	9.8	203.51
Preoperative MOXFQ walking/ standing	47.0		57.6		66.7	
Postoperative MOXFQ walking/ standing	27.6		29.7		40.6	
Difference in MOXFQ walking/ standing	19.4	56.37	27.9	58.92	26.1	70.18
Preoperative MOXFQ social interaction	40.3		55.5		54.0	
Postoperative MOXFQ social interaction	21.8		17.6		35.1	
Difference in MOXFQ social interaction	18.5	59.13	37.9	43.37	18.9	96.9
Preoperative VAS pain	52.2		57.5		57.7	
Postoperative VAS pain	24.5		32.9		13	
Difference in VAS pain	27.5	39.78	24.6	66.83	44.7	40.98
Preoperative EQ5D pain	0.69		0.47		0.48	
Postoperative EQ5D pain	0.74		0.63		0.71	
Difference in EQ5D pain	−0.049	-	0.16	102.74	0.23	79.63

Abbreviations: EQ5D, Euroqol 5D; MOXFQ, Manchester Oxford Foot Questionnaire; VAS, visual analogue score.

surgery, suggesting no improvement or worsening pain after surgery. This could, however, be a type 2 error.

Our study highlights the complexity of examining cost-effectiveness by comparing cost of treatment and improvements in PROM scores. Although significant improvements are demonstrated in PROMS scores there is no significant difference in cost/points. The study is limited in size, additional procedures were not considered in cost, and a difference in indications for each treatment strategy makes direct comparison challenging.

Our study aside, CEA is extremely difficult to perform and equally difficult to compare with other studies. When planning a study there are many variables to consider. There needs to be standardization of the diagnostic criteria for hallux valgus, grading of severity, and treatment algorithms. There needs to be a uniform agreement on measurement of cost-effectiveness. There needs to be consideration of all factors that could influence cost for, for example, inpatient stay, theater, personnel, outpatient reviews, imaging costs, splints, orthotics and dressing costs, the cost of complications, and of course the cost of implants. The cost of implants and use of implants is extremely variable across the globe. In addition, there is also currently little evidence published on the cost-effectiveness of nonoperative treatments for comparison. Perhaps most importantly there needs to also be consideration of the cost of surgery to the patient: if they incur hospital fees and in terms of time out of work and a potential reduction in pay.

SUMMARY

Despite these challenges, there has been, and will remain, a significant increase in health care costs. During times of austerity, greater emphasis has been placed on delivering the most cost-effective health care possible within the constraints of health service budgets. Individual factors influencing cost are more easily studied, with evidence now available that bilateral surgery can reduce cost safely, and that modern regional anesthesia techniques can reduce length of stay, we recommend a pragmatic approach to future cost-effectiveness research.[32,33,36–38]

DISCLOSURE

The authors have nothing to disclose.

REFERENCES

1. Wagner E, Ortiz C, Torres K, et al. Cost effectiveness of different techniques in hallux valgus surgery. Foot Ankle Surg 2016;22(4):259–64.
2. Nix S, Smith M, Vicenzino B. Prevalence of hallux valgus in the general population: a systematic review and meta-analysis. J Foot Ankle Res 2010;3:21.
3. Dunn JE, Link CL, Felson DT, et al. Prevalence of foot and ankle conditions in a multiethnic community sample of older adults. Am J Epidemiol 2004;159:491–8.
4. Abhishek A, Roddy E, Zhang W, et al. Are hallux valgus and big toe pain associated with impaired quality of life? A cross-sectional study. Osteoarthr Cartil 2010; 18-7:923–6.
5. Roddy E, Zhang W, Doherty M. Prevalence and associations of hallux valgus in a primary care population. Arthritis Care Res 2008;59(6):857–62.
6. Green S, Miles R. The burden of disease and illness in the UK: a preliminary assessment to inform the development of UK health research and development priorities. Oxford (MI): Oxford Healthcare Associates; 2007. Version 2.

7. Centers for Medicare and Medicaid Services. National Health Expenditures. 2017. Available at: www.cms.gov. Accessed March 8, 2019.

8. Eurostat Statistics Explained. Healthcare expenditure statistics. 2018. Available at: https://ec.europa.eu/eurostat/statistics-explained/index.php/Healthcare_expenditure_statistics#Health_care_expenditure. Accessed March 8, 2019.

9. Przywara B. European Economy, Economic Papers 417, projecting future health care expenditure at European level: drivers, methodology and main results. Brussels, July 2010.

10. Mickle KJ, Munro BJ, Lord SR, et al. ISB Clinical Biomechanics Award 2009: toe weakness and deformity increase the risk of falls in older people. Clin Biomech (Bristol, Avon) 2009;24-10:787–91.

11. Menz HB, Lord SR. Gait instability in older people with hallux valgus. Foot Ankle Int 2005;26(6):483–9.

12. North West London Collaboration of Clinical Commissioning Groups. Surgery for hallux valgus (bunions). October 2018. 4.1.1. Available at: https://www.hounslowccg.nhs.uk/media/117285/surgery-for-hallux-valgus-bunions-final-v-4-1-1.pdf. Accessed March 8, 2019.

13. Royal College of Surgeons Commissioning Guide. Painful deformed great toe in adults. Available at: https://www.rcseng.ac.uk/-/media/files/rcs/standards-and-research/commissioning/boa–painful-deformed-great-toe-guide-2017.pdf. Accessed March 8, 2019.

14. NHS England Interim Commissioning policy: Bunion surgery. Available at: https://www.england.nhs.uk/commissioning/wp-content/uploads/sites/12/2013/11/N-SC007.pdf. Accessed March 8, 2019.

15. Belatti DA, Phisitkul P. Economic burden of foot and ankle surgery in the US Medicare population. Foot Ankle Int 2014;35(4):334–40.

16. Center for the Evaluation of Value and Risk in Health. Cost effectivenss analysis database. Available at: https://cevr.tuftsmedicalcenter.org/databases. Accessed March 8, 2019.

17. Sanders GD, Neumann PJ, Basu A, et al. Recommendations for conduct, methodological practices, and reporting of cost-effectiveness analyses: second panel on cost-effectiveness in health and medicine. JAMA 2016;316(10):1093–103.

18. PatientProtectionandAffordableCareAct,42 USC§18001 et seq (2010). 111th Congress Public Law 148.

19. Rajan PV, Qudsi RA, Wolf LL, et al. Orthopaedic forum: cost-effectiveness analyses in orthopaedic surgery, raising the bar. J Bone Joint Surg Am 2017; 99(13):e71.

20. Bozic KJ, Morshed S, Silverstein MD, et al. Use of cost-effectiveness analysis to evaluate new technologies in orthopaedics – the case of alternative bearing surfaces in total hip arthroplasty. J Bone Joint Surg Am 2006;88(4):706–14.

21. Garber AM, Weinstein ML, Torrance CW, et al. Theoretical foundations of cost-effectiveness analysis. In: Gold MR, Siegel JE, Russell LB, et al, editors. Cost-effectiveness in health and medicine. New York: Oxford University Press; 1996. p. 25–53.

22. Brauer CA, Rosen AB, Olchanski NV, et al. Cost-utility analyses in orthopaedic surgery. J Bone Joint Surg Am 2005;87(6):1253–9.

23. Karhade AV, Kwon JY. Cost-utility analyses in us orthopaedic foot and ankle surgery. A systematic review. Foot Ankle Spec 2018;11(6):548–52.

24. Baumhauer JF. Ankle arthrodesis versus ankle replacement for ankle arthritis. Clin Orthop Relat Res 2013;471(8):2439–42.

25. Chen L, Lyman S, Do H. Validation of foot and ankle outcome score for hallux valgus. Foot Ankle Int 2012;33:1145–55.
26. SooHoo NF, Shuler M, Fleming LL. Evaluation of the validity of the AOFAS Clinical Rating Systems by correlation to the SF-36. Foot Ankle Int 2003;24(1):50–5.
27. Sutherland JM, Mok J, Liu G, et al. Cost-utility study of the economics of bunion correction surgery. Foot Ankle Int 2019;40(3):336–42.
28. Bettenhausen DA, Cragel M. The offset-V osteotomy with screw fixation: a retrospective evaluation of unilateral versus bilateral surgery. J Foot Ankle Surg 1997; 36(6):418–21.
29. Weil LS. Scarf osteotomy for correction of hallux valgus. Historical perspective, surgical technique and results. Foot Ankle Clin 2000;5(3):559–80.
30. Lee KB, Hur CI, Chung JY, et al. Outcome of unilateral versus simultaneous correction for hallux valgus. Foot Ankle Int 2009;30(2):120–3.
31. Boychenko AV, Solomin LN, Parfeyev SG, et al. Efficacy of bilateral simultaneous hallux valgus correction compared to unilateral. Foot Ankle Int 2015;36(11): 1339–43.
32. Dawson J, Peters M, Jenkinson C, et al. Unilateral versus bilateral same-day surgery outcomes for hallux valgus: an eight year prospective cohort study. Foot Ankle Online J 2012;5(11):2–12.
33. Fridman R, Cain JD, Weil L, et al. Unilateral versus bilateral first ray surgery: a prospective study of 186 consecutive cases–patient satisfaction, cost to society, and complications. Foot Ankle Spec 2009;2(3):123–9.
34. Torres Campos A, Ezquerra Herraneo L, Blanco Rubio N, et al. Cost effectiveness of a hallux valgus day-surgery program. Rev Esp Cir Ortop Traumatol 2013;57(1): 38–44.
35. Torkki M. Academic discussion. Surgery for Hallux Valgus. Studies on cost-effectiveness and timing of treatment. Helsinki (Finland): From the Department of Orthopaedics and Traumatology and Jorvi Hospital Helsinki University Hospital; 2004. ISBN 952-10-1854-2.
36. Torkki M, Malmivaara A, Seitsalo S, et al. Surgery vs orthosis vs watchful waiting for hallux valgus: a randomised controlled trial. JAMA 2001;285(19):2474–80.
37. Murray O, Holt G, McGrory R, et al. Efficacy of outpatient bilateral simultaneous hallux valgus surgery. Orthopedics 2010;33(6):394.
38. Kim BS, Shim DS, Lee JW. Comparison of multi-drug injection versus placebo after hallux valgus surgery. Foot Ankle Int 2011;32(9):856–60.
39. Spruce MC, Bowling FL, Metcalfe SA. A longitudinal study of hallux valgus surgical outcomes using a validated patient centred outcome measure. Foot (Edinb) 2011;21(3):133–7.
40. Brattwal M, Turan I, Jakobsson J. Pain management after elective hallux valgus surgery: a prospective randomized double-blind study comparing etoricoxib and tramadol. Anesthesia 2010;111(2):544–9.
41. Romero EC, Gomez SG, Candel RP, et al. Unilateral versus simultaneous bilateral percutaneous hallux valgus surgery. SM Min Inv Surg 2017;1(1):1001.
42. Oliva F, Longo UG, Maffulli N. Minimally invasive hallux valgus correction. Orthop Clin North Am 2009;40:525–30.
43. Carvalho P, Viana G, Flora M, et al. Percutaneous hallux valgus treatment: unilaterally or bilaterally. Foot Ankle Surg 2016;22(4):248–53.
44. Maffulli N, Longo UG, Marinozzi A, et al. Hallux valgus: effectiveness and safety of minimally invasive surgery. A systematic review. Br Med Bull 2011;97(1): 149–67.

Use of Advanced Weightbearing Imaging in Evaluation of Hallux Valgus

Cesar de Cesar Netto, MD, PhD[a],*, Martinus Richter, MD, PhD[b]

KEYWORDS

- Hallux valgus • Hallux valgus deformity • Bunion • Sesamoids • Weightbearing
- Computed tomography • Weightbearing computed tomography

KEY POINTS

- Weightbearing conventional radiographs provide limited, sectorized, and biased information regarding the complex and 3-dimensional nature of hallux valgus (HV) deformity, leading to potential misinterpretation and poor understanding.
- Cone beam weightbearing computed tomography (WBCT) allows multiplanar 3-dimensional standing weightbearing imaging and a detailed evaluation of HV deformity.
- WBCT allowed demonstration that the hypermobility of the first tarsometatarsal (TMT) joint occurs not only in the sagittal plane with increased dorsiflexion, but also into other planes, with increased inversion and adduction.
- The hypermobility was shown to be present not only at the first TMT joint, but to extend across the whole first ray, involving the first metatarsophalangeal, naviculocuneiform, and talonavicular joints.
- Measurements of pronation deformity in HV using WBCT do not correlate with traditional weightbearing conventional radiograph HV and intermetatarsal angulations. Surgical planning of HV should consider the 3-dimensional pattern of the deformity, and WBCT images should be used when available.

INTRODUCTION

Hallux valgus (HV) consists of a progressive 3-dimensional deformity that includes bone malalignment, hypermobility of the first ray, and imbalance of soft-tissue structures of the midfoot and forefoot.[1–3]

Clinical examination and conventional radiographs are commonly used in the assessment of HV patients, with anteroposterior (AP), lateral, and oblique views forming the core for imaging evaluation.[4] Different angles measured on weightbearing

[a] Department of Orthopedics and Rehabilitation, University of Iowa, 200 Hawkins Drive, Room 01066 JPP, Lower Level, Iowa City, IA 52242, USA; [b] Department for Foot and Ankle Surgery Rummelsberg and Nuremberg, Location Hospital, Rummelsberg, Rummelsberg 71, Schwarzenbruck 90592, Germany
* Corresponding author.
E-mail address: cesar-netto@uiowa.edu

Foot Ankle Clin N Am 25 (2020) 31–45
https://doi.org/10.1016/j.fcl.2019.10.001
foot.theclinics.com

conventional radiographs have been utilized to describe and stage each component of the deformity.

WEIGHTBEARING CONVENTIONAL RADIOGRAPHIC ASSESSMENT OF HALLUX VALGUS DEFORMITY

Hallux Valgus Angle

HV angle describes the amount of transverse plane valgus deviation of the proximal phalanx (PP) of the first toe over the head of the first metatarsal (M1), measured on AP views of weightbearing conventional radiographs (**Fig. 1**). Represented by the angle between the axis of the M1 and the PP of the first toe, it is considered normal if less than 15° of valgus angulation.[5] It takes part of the staging system of the severity of the pathology in mild, moderate, and severe deformities. It is reliably performed with the use of goniometers in conventional radiographs and with computer-assisted measurements in digital radiographs.[6] However, significant variations in values measured were previously demonstrated depending on the anatomic landmarks used.[7]

Hallux Valgus Interphalangeal Angle

HV interphalangeal angle describes the valgus angulation between the axis of the proximal and distal phalanxes of the first toe, measured in the transverse plane.[8] It is also measured on WBCR AP views and is considered normal when below 10°. Increased angulation in the interphalangeal joint (IP) has been shown to represent a considerable amount of the total valgus deformity of the first toe,[9] with adequate measurement reliability.[10,11]

1 to 2 Intermetatarsal Angle

This measures the angulation between the axis of M1 and the second metatarsal (M2) using WBCR AP views, and a value of 9° or more is considered increased and a sign of relative varus deviation of the M1 in the transverse plane (see **Fig. 1**).[4,5] The angle value is also used in the staging system of HV deformity, and the reliability of its

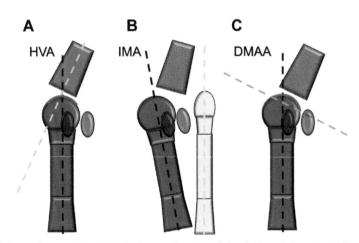

Fig. 1. Hallux valgus angle (HVA) between the axis of the first metatarsal and the proximal phalanx of the first toe (*A*); 1 to 2 intermetatarsal angle (IMA) angulation between the axis of the first and second metatarsals (*B*). Distal metatarsal articular angle (DMAA) measures the angulation between the articular surface of the first metatarsal head and the longitudinal axis of the first metatarsal (*C*).

measurement has been shown to be adequate in the literature,[11] which is more consistent when averaged values of at least 2 readings are used.[12] Significant variation can exist depending on the anatomic landmarks used to define the axis of the metatarsals.[7]

Distal Metatarsal Articular Angle

Distal metatarsal articular angle evaluates the amount valgus angulation between the articular surface and the longitudinal axis of the M1 in the transverse plane, using WBCR AP views (see **Fig. 1**).[13] A value of 7 or less is considered normal. It is the most controversial measurement in the assessment of HV patients, with questions of whether it represents a real entity or just an imaging artifact of conventional radiographs. Measurements have been shown to significantly differ with longitudinal rotation and increased varus of the M1,[14,15] with overall inadequate measurement reliability.[11,16] However, the radiographically measured angle has been shown to significantly correlate with the real anatomic angulation of the articular surface and to be increased in patients with more pronounced deformities.[17]

Sesamoid/Metatarsal Head Positioning

Sesamoid/metatarsal head positioning can be measured in the transverse plane (WBCR AP view) by the evaluation of the relative positioning between the medial sesamoid (MS) and the axis of the M1, grading the amount of lateral displacement and subluxation of the sesamoids. Even though it is known that in the pathophysiological progression of the deformity, the head of M1 deviates medially and pronates, as the sesamoids stay in place connected to an elaborate apparatus of soft tissue structures, to simplify the wording and facilitate understanding, here the term sesamoid displacement/subluxation/dislocation will be used, considering the relative net movement using M1 as the reference point.[3] Seven different degrees of MS positioning were described initially, with grade 1 representing the condition where the lateral edge of the MS is located medially to the axis of the M1; grade 7 represents when the medial edge of the MS is located laterally to it.[5] A simplified 4-stage system using similar landmarks was also described, wherein with grade 0, the MS would be positioned entirely medial for the axial line of the M1. Grade 1 would demonstrate less than 50% overlap of the MS with the line; grade 2 would demonstrate with more than 50% overlap, and grade 3 would be when the MS is located laterally to the axis of the M1 (**Fig. 2**).[18]

Sesamoid positioning can also be measured using in the coronal plane using WBCR standing tangential views. The relative positioning of the MS and the intersesamoid ridge or crista is usually evaluated. Sesamoid subluxation can be graded as the proportion of the MS positioned laterally to the intersesamoid ridge concerning the overall MS width.[18,19] Using that concept, Yildirim and colleagues[20] described a 4-stage classification system, similar to the one used in WBCR AP views. Grade 0 represents the condition where the MS is entirely medial to the intersesamoid crista; grade 1 indicates that less than half the width of the MS is subluxated laterally. Grade 2 shows that more than half the width of the MS is subluxated laterally, and grade 3 indicates that the tibial MS is entirely lateral to the intersesamoid ridge (**Fig. 3**).[20]

Even though measurements of sesamoid positioning using AP and tangential views have been shown to have acceptable reliability in the literature,[19,21] the grading system performed on WBCR AP views demonstrated significant differences when compared with the staging on tangential WBCR views, and to be significantly influenced by the degree of M1 rotation.[18] Different dorsiflexion degrees of the first

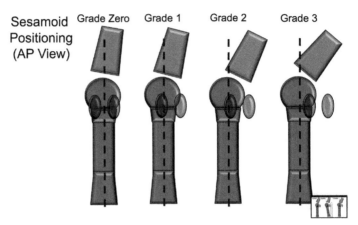

Fig. 2. Four-stage grading system of sesamoid positioning measured on the anteroposterior (AP) view or transverse plane. Considers the relative positioning of the medial sesamoid (MS) to the axis line of the first metatarsal. Grade 0: the MS is positioned entirely medial to the axial line of the M1. Grade 1 demonstrates less than 50% overlap of the MS with the line; Grade 2 with more than 50% overlap, Grade 3 when the MS is located entirely lateral to the axis of the M1.

metatarsophalangeal (MTP) joint at the time of the acquisition of tangential WBCR have also been shown to influence the relative position of the MS, and consequently lead to misclassification on the grading system of sesamoid subluxation.[20] The measurement of the angulation between a line connecting the most plantar aspects of both sesamoid bones and the floor (sesamoid rotation angle – SRA) was reported as a possibly more reliable way of describing sesamoid bone positioning using WBCR standing tangential views (**Fig. 4**).[22]

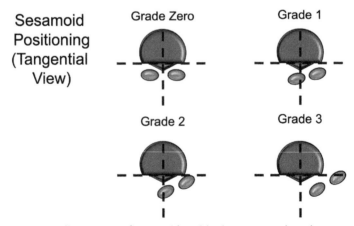

Fig. 3. Four-stage grading system of sesamoid positioning measured on the tangential sesamoid view/coronal plane. Considers the relative positioning of the medial sesamoid (MS) to a bisecting line of the intersesamoid crista. Grade 0: the MS is positioned entirely medial to the line; Grade 1 demonstrates less than 50% overlap of the MS with the line. Grade 2 with more than 50% overlap, and grade 3 when the MS is located entirely lateral to the intersesamoid crista bisecting line.

First Metatarsal and
Sesamoid Rotation
(Tangential
View)

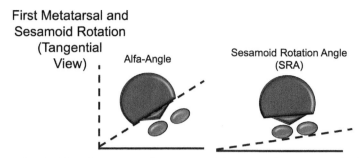

Alfa-Angle

Sesamoid Rotation Angle
(SRA)

Fig. 4. Rotational deformity measured on tangential sesamoid view/coronal plane. First metatarsal rotation angle (alfa angle) measured as the angulation between a line connecting the most inferior medial edge of the medial sesamoid sulcus and the most inferior lateral edge of the lateral sesamoid sulcus and a perpendicular line to the floor. Sesamoid rotation angle (SRA) measured as the angulation between the floor and a tangent line connecting the most inferior aspects of the medial and lateral sesamoids.

M1 Rotation

Measurement is used to grade the amount of pronation of the M1 in the coronal plane that is part of the 3-dimensional HV deformity[23] and thought to be resultant of increased multiplanar motion of the first tarsometatarsal (TMT), naviculocuneiform (NC), and talonavicular (TN) joints.[3,24] M1 rotation is usually measured using WBCR tangential views,[25,26] but descriptions of rotational estimates using WBCR AP views have also reported in the literature, according to the positioning of the inferior tuberosity of the M1 base.[27,28] M1 rotation is measured by the angulation between a line connecting the most inferior medial edge of the medial sesamoid sulcus and the most inferior lateral edge of the lateral sesamoid sulcus and the floor. The angle is positive if pronated and negative if supinated. The angle was found to be reliably performed, demonstrating mean values of pronation in control and HV patients of respectively 1.6° and 5.7°, with a significant 4.3° difference between the groups.[29] More recently, a similar angulation was described as alfa-angle, and was evaluated on simulated WBCT images of HV and control patients (see **Fig. 4**).[30]

LIMITATIONS OF CONVENTIONAL RADIOGRAPHS AND THE RISE OF 3-DIMENSIONAL MULTIPLANAR WEIGHTBEARING IMAGING

Even though conventional radiographs have proven since x-rays were discovered by Wilhelm Conrad Roentgen in 1895, the 2-dimensional nature of this imaging modality in the characterization of complex 3-dimensional deformities is insufficient. Conventional radiographs provide sectorized and limited information of the HV deformity in the different planes, with well-known limitations regarding superimposition of structures, image magnification, x-ray source and patient positioning misalignment, and limited evaluation of rotational deformities. All of these limitations can lead to possible errors during measurement of CR parameters, influencing the variable reliability reported for different HV measures and angulations.[31–33] Recent advances in clinical imaging provided foot and ankle surgeons with new radiological techniques allowing a complete evaluation of complex 3-dimensional deformities.

The advent of computed tomography (CT) allowed a much better evaluation of 3-dimensional components of the osseous anatomy, exposing the patient to a considerable radiation dosage.[34–36] However, although conventional radiographs allow WB and the study of the foot and ankle in a standing, loaded, and physiologic condition, conventional CT was limited to NWB images, limiting the assessment of real relative bone positioning. Attempts have been made in the literature to simulate WB in patients undergoing foot and ankle conventional CT imaging. Most of them include some device that creates a passive compression load force in the lower extremity, without proper and physiologic activation of agonist and antagonist musculature, potentially influencing the positioning of the bones of the foot and ankle.[37–40]

An important advancement has been the introduction of cone beam weightbearing CT (CB WBCT), which allows multiplanar 3-dimensional standing weightbearing bone imaging, with significantly lower radiation doses when compared with conventional CT images, and a detailed evaluation of complex foot and ankle disorders.[32,41–44] The literature on standing WBCT has been growing significantly during the last 5 years.[44–46] Most of it related to the evaluation of another complex 3-dimensional pathology, the adult acquired flatfoot deformity, allowing assessment of the multiple components of the deformity in both 2-dimensional and 3-dimensional images, with overall good to excellent measurement reliability, supporting treatment decision and surgical planning, and currently considered by many authors as part of the gold-standard assessment for patients preoperatively.[47–53]

WEIGHTBEARING CONE BEAM COMPUTED TOMOGRAPHY AND HALLUX VALGUS DEFORMITY

Collan and colleagues[54] were the first to report on the use of standing CB WBCT in the assessment of HV patients. They evaluated 10 patients with HV deformity and 5 controls. Patients underwent resting NWB and standing WB CBCT. They measured 2-dimensional and 3-dimensional HVA and IMA, as well as the rotational status of the M1 and PP of the first toe, using coronal plane images. They found that, when compared with controls, patients with HV deformity demonstrated significantly increased HVA (35° vs 13°; and 35° vs 15°) and IMA (19° vs 11°; and 17° vs 11°) for both 2-dimensional and 3-dimensional WB images, respectively.

The authors also found that 3-dimensional HVA was more pronounced in NWB images when compared with the ones measured during WB, but the differences between HV and control patients did not reach statistical significance. Regarding rotational status, they reported statistically insignificant increased pronation of the M1 in HV patients (8°) compared with controls (2°). However, the PP of the first toe was found to have significant pronation when compared with controls (33° vs 4°). Finally, they reported an excellent correlation between measurements performed on 2-dimensional and 3-dimensional images for both HVA (Pearson = 0.94) and IMA (Pearson = 0.81). The authors concluded that 3-dimensional WBCT could be used in isolation to evaluate patients with HV deformity, providing all relevant data needed, including the rotational component of the deformity.

Geng and colleagues[55] performed a multiplanar analysis of the first TMT joint motion when comparing unloaded and loaded conditions, using simulated WBCT. They included 10 patients with HV deformity and 10 healthy controls. Three-dimensional images of the M1 and medial cuneiform in unloaded condition were matched to the equivalent bones in a loaded condition. The authors found that, when compared with controls, the feet of HV patients demonstrated significant first TMT joint dorsiflexion (average of 2.9° vs 1.2° in controls), supination (average of 2.2° vs 1° in controls), and internal rotation (average 2.6° vs 1° in controls). Interestingly, even though both medial cuneiform and M1 demonstrated increased overpronation since there was more pronounced pronation in the medial cuneiform when compared with the M1, the resultant motion at the first TMT joint was supination. HV patients also presented with significant widening of the first TMT joint, with a trend for increased translation in the dorsal-plantar direction. The authors highlighted the presence of multiplanar and multidirectional hypermobility of the first TMT joint in HV, when assessed by simulated WBCT images, and emphasized that a better understanding of the normal and pathologic 3-dimensional mobility of the joint with this imaging modality could potentially help in the assessment and treatment of HV deformity.

In a similarly designed study, Kimura and colleagues[56] compared relative multiplanar movement of the first ray bones in 10 patients with HV deformity and 10 controls. They found that HV patients demonstrated significantly increased dorsiflexion at the TN joint; eversion and abduction at the NC joint; dorsiflexion, inversion, and adduction at the first TMT joint; and eversion and abduction at the first MTP joint. They also found robust correlations between measurements of HVA and IMA on conventional radiographs and 3-dimensional WBCT images (r = 0.873–0.981). The authors emphasized that simulated WBCT allowed demonstration of increased hypermobility of the first TMT joint, not only in the sagittal plane with increased dorsiflexion, but also into other planes, with increased inversion and adduction. More than that, they also highlighted that the hypermobility extends across the entire first ray, with the involvement of multiple other joints. They suggested that the assessment and the treatment plan of HV patients should also be addressed in 3 dimensions.

The same authors compared the relative 3-dimensional movement between the 3 cuneiform bones between the middle cuneiform and the navicular using simulated WBCT.[57] They included 11 patients with HV and 11 controls. They found that under load and relative to the medial cuneiform, the middle cuneiform demonstrated significantly increased dorsiflexion and inversion in HV patients when compared with controls. No significant differences were found for the relative positioning in between the middle and lateral cuneiforms, as well as the middle cuneiform and the navicular bone. They concluded that HV deformity is also associated with hypermobility of the joint between the medial and middle cuneiforms, hypothesizing that this joint should be potentially stabilized in patients with severe first ray hypermobility.

Kim and colleagues[30] used simulated WBCT to evaluate the role of axial plane CT images in the assessment of HV and metatarsosesamoid rotational deformities and sesamoid bone positioning. The authors compared simulated WBCT and conventional measurements of 138 HV patients and 19 controls. They found that the alfa-angle, measuring the rotational deformity of the M1 in pronation, to be significantly increased in HV patients (21.9°) when compared with controls (13.8°). A weak positive correlation was found between the alfa-angle and other measures performed, including HVA, IMA, and the degree of sesamoid subluxation. Using the control group to define a trustful confidence interval of normal M1 rotation, the authors found that 87.3% of the HV feet studied demonstrated significantly increased alfa-angle, or in other words, 87.3% had significant pronation deformity. The authors highlighted the possibility of misleading pseudo-sesamoid subluxation when using WBCR AP views and the 7-grade classification system of sesamoid displacement.[5] More specifically, they showed that 25.9% of the HV patients had increased lateral deviation on AP WBCR images and M1 pronation on simulated WBCT axial plane images, but no real subluxation of the sesamoid from its articular facet, when using the 4-grade system classification of sesamoid subluxation.[18–20] These findings emphasize the potential misinterpretation and misclassification of sesamoid subluxation when using WBCR images and a complete assessment of the deformity when using WBCT. A weak positive correlation was found between the alfa-angle and HVA, IMA, and the degree of sesamoid subluxation. The authors also proposed a new classification system for

HV deformity, based on WBCT axial images evaluation, that divides the patients into 4 different groups depending upon findings of presence or absence of increased M1 pronation (threshold value of more than 15.8°) and sesamoid bone subluxation (threshold value equal or superior to grade 1).

Campbell and colleagues[58] quantified 3 dimensionally the pronation deformities of M1 relative to the M2 and the PP of the first toe in relation to the M1. They included 10 HV patients and 10 controls who underwent simulated WBCT and WBCR. The authors encountered a significant difference averaging 8.2° of increased pronation of M1 and 14.5° of first toe pronation when comparing HV patients and controls. The severity of M1 and first toe pronation 3-dimensional measurements on simulated WBCT images were not predicted by the WBCR measurements of IMA or HVA angulation. There was also no significant correlation between the amount of first toe and M1 3-dimensional pronation, suggesting that the deformities should be assessed and considered independently. The authors concluded that pronation represents an important deformity component of HV and that surgical treatment planning should consider the multiplanar pattern of the deformity. They cautioned the risks of using WBCR 2-dimensional measurements such as HVA and IMA as surgical planning tools, endangering inadequate understanding of the deformity and poor treatment options.

Welck and colleagues[59] investigated the position of the sesamoid bones, their rotation, and the metatarsosesamoid joint space using standing CB WBCT in 43 patients with symptomatic HV and compared the results with a group of 50 control patients. Aiming to measure sesamoid positioning, the authors used the coronal plane section where the crista was most prominent or the image where the widest portion of the M1 head was noted, when the crista was eroded entirely. HVA, IMA, SRA, and a 4-stage positioning of the sesamoid bones were measured. They found high intra- and interobserver reliabilities for all measurements, ranging from 0.96 to 1.00, and demonstrated significantly increased HVA (33.8° vs 11.7°), IMA (16.9° vs 10.7°), SRA (29.2° vs 9.7°), and sesamoid displacement (1.58 vs 0.04) in HV patients when compared with controls. The shortest distance between the medial sesamoid articular surface and the opposing M1 head, measured in millimeters, was found to be significantly decreased in HV patients (0.42 mm vs 1.29 mm). In the same study, the authors proposed a new classification system for sesamoid bone positioning using standing WBCT findings for HV patients, the Stanmore Classification System, which would consider the positioning and the amount of sesamoid wear. Degeneration of the metatarsosesamoid joint was graded as (A) normal (joint space higher than 1 mm), (B) reduced (joint space of less than 1 mm), (C) absent (bone on bone), and with (D) bone destruction (determined by an empty intersesamoid crista). Sesamoid positioning was measured in a 4-stage system (0, 1, 2, 3, and 4), as previously described in the literature.[19] The authors concluded that standing WBCT imaging allowed accurate and reproducible assessment of relative sesamoid displacement and metatarsosesamoid joint space narrowing in patients with HV. In their opinion, the 3-dimensional assessment of the sesamoid bones preoperatively using the proposed classification system can potentially influence the surgical decision making, helping in the treatment of HV patients. However, the authors emphasize that future prognostic and prospective studies are needed.

WEIGHTBEARING COMPUTED TOMOGRAPHY ARTIFICIAL INTELLIGENCE AND AUTOMATIC MEASUREMENTS: THE NEXT STEP

The recently published literature demonstrates that WBCT measurements provide a complete analysis of all 3-dimensional components of the HV deformity. However, the amount of data acquired during the examination is vast and can represent a burden, needing a critical amount of time and effort for adequate interpretation. The more accurate 3-dimensional measurements usually include the need for a manual or semiautomatic segmentation of each tarsal bone involved in the measure, using different surface or volume landmarks. The advent of artificial intelligence (AI) and automatic segmentation and measurement tools would represent a crucial advance in the assessment of HV and other complex foot deformities.

AI-based automatic measurement tools are currently based on machine learning, which requires the lengthy and painstaking process of training algorithms to accomplish a given task by feeding it with enormous quantities of data. In the case of measurements in the forefoot, in particular for HV deformity, this requires first for the software to correctly identify the first and second metatarsals and completely differentiate them from surrounding bones. This is technically challenging, especially around the base of the M2 and in the first MTP joint, where arthritic changes often occur in association with HV. Also, the presence of metalwork does not allow the software to function normally. In that case, the software does not produce a value. Nevertheless, with the collaboration of the industry recent advances allowed the authors, within the International Weight Bearing CT Society (https://www.wbctsociety.org), to perform a preliminary investigation of this new generation tool. At the time this article was written, for which three centers collaborated, the AI software was able to produce measurements successfully from 59% to 95% of cases.

In order to evaluate an AI-based automatic measurement tool (Automatic IMA, Cubeview, Curvebeam, Hattfield Pennsylvania), the authors evaluated intraobserver or in this case intrasoftware reproducibility (the observer is the software itself) of AI automatic measurements performed by the software compared with human measurements performed by themselves. The objective was to investigate whether the reproducibility of AI-based measurements of the IMA was superior to human measurements in a group of 12 patients with HV deformity and 12 healthy controls. Exclusion criteria were a history of forefoot surgery involving the first or second metatarsals, the presence of metalwork anywhere in the foot and ankle, cases of severe arthritis of the first MTP joint, and failure of the AI software to produce a measurement.

All patients underwent a bilateral standing WBCT using a PedCAT unit (CurveBeam LLC, 175 Titus Ave, Suite 300, Warrington, Pennsylvania). The datasets were extracted from the existing database, containing the 3-dimensional image data and the demographics of the patients including age, sex, and body mass index (BMI). Measurements were made twice, independently by a fellowship trained senior foot and ankle orthopedic surgeon and a trained research assistant. The IMA measurements were made by hand using the available software tools (simple Cobb angle measurements) on the digitally reconstructed radiographs (DRR) produced by the standard WBCT software (**Fig. 5**). The AI produces a 3-dimensional IMA (**Fig. 6**) and a 2-dimensional IMA, which is the projection of the former onto the ground plane, mimicking the angle that is traditionally obtained on a conventional radiograph. Statistics were performed independently by a third investigator. The demographic data and the IMA were compared using a 1-way ANOVA test and significance assessed using a rank sums test. Intraobserver intraclass correlation (ICC) coefficients were calculated for both human observers and the AI software. Interobserver ICCs could only be calculated for the 2o human observers, since only 1 AI software was used for this pilot study.

The authors found in this preliminary study that HV cases were significantly older than controls (mean 62.9 vs 43.8, $P<.005$). BMI was not significantly different. The mean IMA manually measured on DRR was 13.6 (12.9–14.3) in HV patients versus

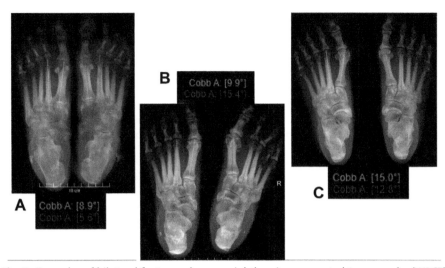

Fig. 5. Examples of bilateral feet cone beam weightbearing computed tomography (WBCT) manual measurements of 1 to 2 IMA performed on digitally reconstructed radiographs (DRR). Control (*A*) and HV patients (*B*, *C*). Top measurements for the left foot and bottom measurements for the right foot.

9.0 (8.4–9.70) in controls (*P*<.0001). The mean 2-dimensional IMA measured by the AI was 13.1 (12.0–14.3) for HV cases versus 9.6 (8.5–10.7) in controls. The intraobserver ICCs were 0.65 and 0.8 respectively in controls and HV cases for human observers and manual measurements. The intrasoftware ICC coefficients of the AI for both 2-dimensional and 3-dimensional angles, in controls and HV cases, were all equal to 1 or very close. The interobserver ICCs of human observers were respectively 0.81 and 0.86 for controls and HV cases. These preliminary results show interesting

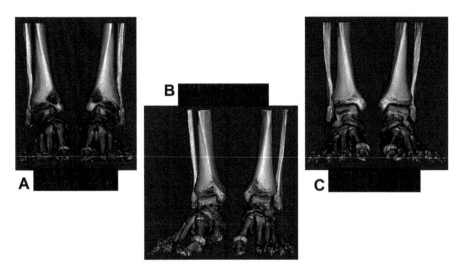

Fig. 6. Examples of bilateral feet automatic 3-dimensional cone beam WBCT measurements of 1 to 2 IMA. Control (*A*) and HV patients (*B*, *C*). Top measurements for the left foot and bottom measurements for the right foot.

potential for AI-based automatic measurement systems using WBCT data in HV deformity. The software seems faster and more reliable than people. However, the success rate of the preliminary bone segmentation process required to perform the IMA measurements is still insufficient to allow implementation in the clinical setting.

SUMMARY AND FUTURE PERSPECTIVES

The pieces of evidence in the orthopedic literature supporting the use of CB WBCT imaging in the assessment of different complex deformities of the foot and ankle has been growing consistently.[44–47,59–63] It is the author's opinion that standing CB WBCT will soon represent the gold standard imaging evaluation of foot and ankle pathologies, replacing WBCR. It is clear that the WBCR assessment of multiplanar pathologies is limited by multiple biases related to acquisition and interpretation of superimposed and distorted uniplanar images, hindering the understanding of all components of multifaceted deformities, and potentially limiting the thinking and the discussion of new treatment options as well as the development of new and more accurate corrective surgical techniques.

Regarding HV deformity, the literature to date on the use of CB WBCT imaging is still scarce. Prospective and outcome studies are needed. However, it already demonstrates important advances that include the ability to reliably perform traditional measurements such as HVA and IMA in the 3-dimensional setting, as well as a more complete and accurate evaluation of the deformity, allowing a better understanding of the multiplanar relative positioning of the bones of the first and second rays.[30,54–59]

The use of AI in the interpretation of CB WBCT data, development of semiautomatic and automatic measurements,[64] integration of plantar pressure data[65] and articular distance mapping,[66] progress of surgical planning tools, and custom-made guides and implants[67] for the treatment of HV deformity represent developments to be explored in the near future.

The use of 2-dimensional imaging in the evaluation of HV and other complex deformities of the foot and ankle is antiquated. One should embrace new technologies and accept that things change. It is in the best interest of patients, who are continually looking for more precise diagnostics, detailed explanations, surgical planning, and improved outcomes. Rest in peace, conventional radiographs!

DISCLOSURE

Dr C. de Cesar Netto reports paid consultancy and share options for CurveBeam LLC, as well as paid consultancy for Ossio LTD. Dr C. de Cesar Netto is also a board member of the International Weight-Bearing CT Society. Dr M. Richter reports paid consultancy for CurveBeam LLC, Ossio LTD, Geistlich, and Intercus. He is also proprietor of R-Innovation and the current president of the International Weight-Bearing CT Society.

REFERENCES

1. Dietze A, Bahlke U, Martin H, et al. First ray instability in hallux valgus deformity: a radiokinematic and pedobarographic analysis. Foot Ankle Int 2013;34(1):124–30.
2. Voellmicke KV, Deland JT. Manual examination technique to assess dorsal instability of the first ray. Foot Ankle Int 2002;23(11):1040–1.
3. Perera AM, Mason L, Stephens MM. The pathogenesis of hallux valgus. J Bone Joint Surg Am 2011;93(17):1650–61.

4. Mann RA, Coughlin MJ. Hallux valgus–etiology, anatomy, treatment and surgical considerations. Clin Orthop Relat Res 1981;(157):31–41.

5. Hardy RH, Clapham JC. Observations on hallux valgus; based on a controlled series. J Bone Joint Surg Br 1951;33-B(3):376–91.

6. Farber DC, Deorio JK, Steel MW 3rd. Goniometric versus computerized angle measurement in assessing hallux valgus. Foot Ankle Int 2005;26(3):234–8.

7. Schneider W, Knahr K. Metatarsophalangeal and intermetatarsal angle: different values and interpretation of postoperative results dependent on the technique of measurement. Foot Ankle Int 1998;19(8):532–6.

8. Mann RA. Disorders of the First Metatarsophalangeal Joint. J Am Acad Orthop Surg 1995;3(1):34–43.

9. Strydom A, Saragas NP, Ferrao PN. A radiographic analysis of the contribution of hallux valgus interphalangeus to the total valgus deformity of the hallux. Foot Ankle Surg 2017;23(1):27–31.

10. Hujazi I, Yassa R, Sevenoaks H, et al. Hallux valgus interphalangeus: reliability of radiological assessment. Foot Ankle Surg 2018;25(4):507–10.

11. Coughlin MJ, Freund E. Roger A. Mann Award. The reliability of angular measurements in hallux valgus deformities. Foot Ankle Int 2001;22(5):369–79.

12. Condon F, Kaliszer M, Conhyea D, et al. The first intermetatarsal angle in hallux valgus: an analysis of measurement reliability and the error involved. Foot Ankle Int 2002;23(8):717–21.

13. Mitchell LA, Baxter DE. A Chevron-Akin double osteotomy for correction of hallux valgus. Foot Ankle 1991;12(1):7–14.

14. Vittetoe DA, Saltzman CL, Krieg JC, et al. Validity and reliability of the first distal metatarsal articular angle. Foot Ankle Int 1994;15(10):541–7.

15. Robinson AH, Cullen NP, Chhaya NC, et al. Variation of the distal metatarsal articular angle with axial rotation and inclination of the first metatarsal. Foot Ankle Int 2006;27(12):1036–40.

16. Chi TD, Davitt J, Younger A, et al. Intra- and inter-observer reliability of the distal metatarsal articular angle in adult hallux valgus. Foot Ankle Int 2002;23(8):722–6.

17. Jastifer JR, Coughlin MJ, Schutt S, et al. Comparison of radiographic and anatomic distal metatarsal articular angle in cadaver feet. Foot Ankle Int 2014; 35(4):389–93.

18. Talbot KD, Saltzman CL. Assessing sesamoid subluxation: how good is the AP radiograph? Foot Ankle Int 1998;19(8):547–54.

19. Smith RW, Reynolds JC, Stewart MJ. Hallux valgus assessment: report of research committee of American Orthopaedic Foot and Ankle Society. Foot Ankle 1984;5(2):92–103.

20. Yildirim Y, Cabukoglu C, Erol B, et al. Effect of metatarsophalangeal joint position on the reliability of the tangential sesamoid view in determining sesamoid position. Foot Ankle Int 2005;26(3):247–50.

21. Saltzman CL, Brandser EA, Berbaum KS, et al. Reliability of standard foot radiographic measurements. Foot Ankle Int 1994;15(12):661–5.

22. Kuwano T, Nagamine R, Sakaki K, et al. New radiographic analysis of sesamoid rotation in hallux valgus: comparison with conventional evaluation methods. Foot Ankle Int 2002;23(9):811–7.

23. Hicks JH. The mechanics of the foot. I. The joints. J Anat 1953;87(4):345–57.

24. Saffo G, Wooster MF, Stevens M, et al. First metatarsocuneiform joint arthrodesis: a five-year retrospective analysis. J Foot Surg 1989;28(5):459–65.

25. Inman VT. Hallux valgus: a review of etiologic factors. Orthop Clin North Am 1974; 5(1):59–66.

26. Kay DB, Njus G, Parrish W, et al. Basilar crescentic osteotomy. A three-dimensional computer simulation. Orthop Clin North Am 1989;20(4):571–82.

27. Eustace S, Byrne JO, Beausang O, et al. Hallux valgus, first metatarsal pronation and collapse of the medial longitudinal arch–a radiological correlation. Skeletal Radiol 1994;23(3):191–4.

28. Eustace S, O'Byrne J, Stack J, et al. Radiographic features that enable assessment of first metatarsal rotation: the role of pronation in hallux valgus. Skeletal Radiol 1993;22(3):153–6.

29. Saltzman CL, Brandser EA, Anderson CM, et al. Coronal plane rotation of the first metatarsal. Foot Ankle Int 1996;17(3):157–61.

30. Kim Y, Kim JS, Young KW, et al. A new measure of tibial sesamoid position in hallux valgus in relation to the coronal rotation of the first metatarsal in CT Scans. Foot Ankle Int 2015;36(8):944–52.

31. Willauer P, Sangeorzan BJ, Whittaker EC, et al. The sensitivity of standard radiographic foot measures to misalignment. Foot Ankle Int 2014;35(12):1334–40.

32. Richter M, Seidl B, Zech S, et al. PedCAT for 3D-imaging in standing position allows for more accurate bone position (angle) measurement than radiographs or CT. Foot Ankle Surg 2014;20(3):201–7.

33. Baverel L, Brilhault J, Odri G, et al. Influence of lower limb rotation on hindfoot alignment using a conventional two-dimensional radiographic technique. Foot Ankle Surg 2017;23(1):44–9.

34. Ambrose J. Computerized transverse axial scanning (tomography). 2. Clinical application. Br J Radiol 1973;46(552):1023–47.

35. Ambrose J, Hounsfield G. Computerized transverse axial tomography. Br J Radiol 1973;46(542):148–9.

36. Perry BJ, Bridges C. Computerized transverse axial scanning (tomography). 3. Radiation dose considerations. Br J Radiol 1973;46(552):1048–51.

37. Ananthakrisnan D, Ching R, Tencer A, et al. Subluxation of the talocalcaneal joint in adults who have symptomatic flatfoot. J Bone Joint Surg Am 1999;81(8):1147–54.

38. Malicky ES, Crary JL, Houghton MJ, et al. Talocalcaneal and subfibular impingement in symptomatic flatfoot in adults. J Bone Joint Surg Am 2002;84-A(11):2005–9.

39. Ferri M, Scharfenberger AV, Goplen G, et al. Weightbearing CT scan of severe flexible pes planus deformities. Foot Ankle Int 2008;29(2):199–204.

40. Kido M, Ikoma K, Imai K, et al. Load response of the tarsal bones in patients with flatfoot deformity: in vivo 3D study. Foot Ankle Int 2011;32(11):1017–22.

41. Carrino JA, Al Muhit A, Zbijewski W, et al. Dedicated cone-beam CT system for extremity imaging. Radiology 2014;270(3):816–24.

42. Hirschmann A, Pfirrmann CW, Klammer G, et al. Upright cone CT of the hindfoot: comparison of the non-weight-bearing with the upright weight-bearing position. Eur Radiol 2014;24(3):553–8.

43. Richter M, Zech S, Hahn S, et al. Combination of pedCAT(R) for 3D imaging in standing position with pedography shows no statistical correlation of bone position with force/pressure distribution. J Foot Ankle Surg 2016;55(2):240–6.

44. Barg A, Bailey T, Richter M, et al. Weightbearing computed tomography of the foot and ankle: emerging technology topical review. Foot Ankle Int 2018;39(3):376–86.

45. Lintz F, de Cesar Netto C, Barg A, et al. Weight-bearing cone beam CT scans in the foot and ankle. EFORT Open Rev 2018;3(5):278–86.

46. Godoy-Santos AL, Cesar CN, Weight-Bearing CT International Study Group. Weight-bearing computed tomography of the foot and ankle: an update and future directions. Acta Ortop Bras 2018;26(2):135–9.

47. de Cesar Netto C, Schon LC, Thawait GK, et al. Flexible adult acquired flatfoot deformity: comparison between weight-bearing and non-weight-bearing measurements using cone-beam computed tomography. J Bone Joint Surg Am 2017;99(18):e98.

48. Kunas GC, Probasco W, Haleem AM, et al. Evaluation of peritalar subluxation in adult acquired flatfoot deformity using computed tomography and weightbearing multiplanar imaging. Foot Ankle Surg 2018;24(6):495–500.

49. Burssens A, Van Herzele E, Leenders T, et al. Weightbearing CT in normal hindfoot alignment - Presence of a constitutional valgus? Foot Ankle Surg 2018;24(3):213–8.

50. de Cesar Netto C, Shakoor D, Roberts L, et al. Hindfoot alignment of adult acquired flatfoot deformity: A comparison of clinical assessment and weightbearing cone beam CT examinations. Foot Ankle Surg 2018. [Epub ahead of print].

51. de Cesar Netto C, Shakoor D, Dein EJ, et al. Influence of investigator experience on reliability of adult acquired flatfoot deformity measurements using weightbearing computed tomography. Foot Ankle Surg 2019;25(4):495–502.

52. Peiffer M, Belvedere C, Clockaerts S, et al. Three-dimensional displacement after a medializing calcaneal osteotomy in relation to the osteotomy angle and hindfoot alignment. Foot Ankle Surg 2018. [Epub ahead of print].

53. Burssens A, Barg A, van Ovost E, et al. The hind- and midfoot alignment computed after a medializing calcaneal osteotomy using a 3D weightbearing CT. Int J Comput Assist Radiol Surg 2019;14(8):1439–47.

54. Collan L, Kankare JA, Mattila K. The biomechanics of the first metatarsal bone in hallux valgus: a preliminary study utilizing a weight bearing extremity CT. Foot Ankle Surg 2013;19(3):155–61.

55. Geng X, Wang C, Ma X, et al. Mobility of the first metatarsal-cuneiform joint in patients with and without hallux valgus: in vivo three-dimensional analysis using computerized tomography scan. J Orthop Surg Res 2015;10:140.

56. Kimura T, Kubota M, Taguchi T, et al. Evaluation of first-ray mobility in patients with hallux valgus using weight-bearing CT and a 3-D analysis system: a comparison with normal feet. J Bone Joint Surg Am 2017;99(3):247–55.

57. Kimura T, Kubota M, Suzuki N, et al. Comparison of intercuneiform 1-2 joint mobility between hallux valgus and normal feet using weightbearing computed tomography and 3-dimensional analysis. Foot Ankle Int 2018;39(3):355–60.

58. Campbell B, Miller MC, Williams L, et al. Pilot study of a 3-dimensional method for analysis of pronation of the first metatarsal of hallux valgus patients. Foot Ankle Int 2018;39(12):1449–56.

59. Welck MJ, Singh D, Cullen N, et al. Evaluation of the 1st metatarso-sesamoid joint using standing CT - The Stanmore classification. Foot Ankle Surg 2018;24(4):314–9.

60. Lawlor MC, Kluczynski MA, Marzo JM. Weight-bearing cone-beam CT scan assessment of stability of supination external rotation ankle fractures in a cadaver model. Foot Ankle Int 2018;39(7):850–7.

61. Shakoor D, Osgood GM, Brehler M, et al. Cone-beam CT measurements of distal tibio-fibular syndesmosis in asymptomatic uninjured ankles: does weight-bearing matter? Skeletal Radiol 2019;48(4):583–94.

62. Patel S, Malhotra K, Cullen NP, et al. Defining reference values for the normal tibiofibular syndesmosis in adults using weight-bearing CT. Bone Joint J 2019;101-B(3):348–52.

63. Cheung ZB, Myerson MS, Tracey J, et al. Weightbearing CT scan assessment of foot alignment in patients with hallux rigidus. Foot Ankle Int 2018;39(1):67–74.
64. Lintz F, Welck M, Bernasconi A, et al. 3D biometrics for hindfoot alignment using weightbearing CT. Foot Ankle Int 2017;38(6):684–9.
65. Richter M, Lintz F, Zech S, et al. Combination of PedCAT weightbearing CT with pedography assessment of the relationship between anatomy-based foot center and force/pressure-based center of gravity. Foot Ankle Int 2018;39(3):361–8.
66. Siegler S, Konow T, Belvedere C, et al. Analysis of surface-to-surface distance mapping during three-dimensional motion at the ankle and subtalar joints. J Biomech 2018;76:204–11.
67. Berlet GC, Penner MJ, Lancianese S, et al. Total Ankle Arthroplasty Accuracy and Reproducibility Using Preoperative CT Scan-Derived, Patient-Specific Guides. Foot Ankle Int 2014;35(7):665–76.

Current Trends in Anesthesia Management in Hallux Valgus

Max Seiter, MD[a], Amiethab Aiyer, MD[b],*

KEYWORDS

- Anesthesia • Hallux valgus • Analgesia • Foot and ankle • Multimodal • Nerve block
- Pain

KEY POINTS

- Hallux valgus correction, including bilateral cases, is trending toward outpatient surgery. Multimodal anesthesia/analgesia facilitates this goal, maximizing pain control and minimizing unwanted side effects.
- This approach includes locoregional anesthesia and perioperative intravenous/oral medications: nonsteroidal anti-inflammatory drugs, acetaminophen, gabapentin, opioid agonists, steroids, and N-methyl-D-aspartate agonists, among others.
- Multimodal anesthesia has been proven to optimize pain control, enhance patient satisfaction, and reduce requirement on opiate medications, as well as reduce readmissions for pain.

INTRODUCTION

Modern anesthesia in hallux valgus surgery is focused on multimodal analgesia, enabling better pain control, earlier mobilization, and fewer side effects or complications, as well as decreasing reliance on opiate medications. All of these factors facilitate successful outpatient care. An over-reliance on narcotic medication for pain control has contributed to the current opioid epidemic and has been associated with inferior outcomes after surgery.[1] Accordingly there has been a resurgence of interest in alternative interventions for pain control.

Multimodal treatment consists of a combination of perioperative analgesic medications (anti-inflammatories, opiate agonists, neuromodulatory medications, steroids, and others), plus locoregional anesthesia techniques, such as neuraxial anesthesia, peripheral nerve blocks, or wound infiltration with anesthetics. The use of regional anesthesia is preferred over general; it avoids traditional side effects of general

[a] Sports Medicine Orthopaedic Surgery, Steadman Philippon Research Institute, 181 W Meadow Dr., Vail, CO 81657, USA; [b] Orthopaedic Surgery, University of Miami, Jackson Memorial Hospital, 900 NW 17th Street, Miami, FL 33136, USA
* Corresponding author.
E-mail address: Tabsaiyer@gmail.com

anesthetics and sedative or narcotic medications, and maximizes poor postoperative pain control and mobility, which are obstacles to successful outpatient surgery.[2] The safety and efficacy of regional anesthesia, such as a popliteal nerve block, has been demonstrated in numerous studies, including level 1 evidence from randomized, controlled trials showing minimal complications, good pain control, and high patient satisfaction.[3–7]

The culmination into a multimodal analgesia program has further improved patient outcomes in hallux valgus surgery and across orthopedics as a whole, with decreased length of hospitalization, decreased opioid use and adverse effects, better pain scores, and earlier rehabilitation.[7–10] These advances in acute and postoperative pain management have normalized hallux valgus correction as an outpatient procedure, feasible even in patients undergoing bilateral surgery, who were traditionally relegated to inpatient admission owing to concerns about pain control.[3,11]

Increased postoperative pain is associated with an increase in complications; patients with increased pain even on the first day after surgery may show a 2-fold increase in complications after orthopedic procedures.[12] Increased postoperative pain after hallux valgus surgery has been shown to result in higher readmission rates, prolonged hospital stays, higher cost of care, and slower overall recovery.[13–15]

Analgesic medications categories include nonsteroidal anti-inflammatory drugs (NSAIDs; namely, cyclooxygenase [COX]-1 and -2 inhibitors), acetaminophen, neuromodulatory medications (gabapentin, pregabalin), opioid agonists, combined opioid agonist-selective serotonin/norepinephrine reuptake inhibitors (tramadol, tapentadol), glucocorticoids, and N-methyl-D-aspartate antagonists (ketamine, memantine); the mechanisms of actions, dosing, positive features, and side effects of each drug are listed in **Table 1**.

Several level one studies have demonstrated improved pain relief when examining the effects of acetaminophen, NSAIDs, COX-2 selective inhibitors, opioids, and intravenous (IV) dexamethasone; evidenced by reduced opioid intake and improved pain scores.

ANALGESIC MEDICATIONS

NSAIDs include COX-1 and COX-2 inhibitors COX-2 specific inhibitors in both oral and IV formulations. In a randomized controlled trial of 100 patients undergoing hallux valgus surgery, Brattwall and colleagues[16] compared the use of etorcoxib and tramadol in the immediate 7-day postoperative period. Patients receiving the NSAID displayed decreased pain in the 1-week period after surgery, increased satisfaction rates, and decreased side effects when compared with tramadol, without signs of increased wound complications or impaired bony healing at 12 week follow-up.

Acetaminophen

Perioperative use of acetaminophen has consistently demonstrated a synergistic effect on pain management when used in concert with both regional anesthesia and NSAIDs.[9,17,18]

Opioid Agonists

Although narcotics carry well-documented risks and negative side effects, they remain central to the armamentarium of perioperative pain control, particularly for breakthrough or escape pain. The opioid epidemic must be considered and, as such, all other modalities for pain control should be used, minimizing reliance on opiate medications.

Table 1
Medications available for use in multimodal anesthesia; all listed categories of medications may be used concurrently

Medication	Mechanism of Action	Dosing	Positive Features	Side Effects/Complications
NSAIDs				
Ibuprofen, naproxen, diclofenac, indomethacin, meloxicam (PO)	COX-1 and -2 inhibitor (nonspecific)	400–800 mg q6h	No addictive potential, OTC, efficacious analgesic	Potential renal toxicity, platelet inhibition, inhibition of bone and soft tissue healing, gastric mucosa effects
Ketorolac (IV)		15–30 mg q6h (limit 6 doses total)	Potent analgesic	Cardiovascular risk, gastric mucosa effects, higher gastric mucosa toxicity compared with other NSAIDs
Celecoxib	COX-2 inhibitor (specific)	200 mg q12h	Reduced platelet effect, reduced gastric toxicity	Increased cardiovascular risk, potential renal toxicity
Acetaminophen	CNS inhibition of COX, modulation of central serotonin		Well tolerated	Caution with hepatic disease
Acetaminophen (PO)		Up to 1 g q6h	Inexpensive	May not produce therapeutic levels in perioperative period
Paracetamol (IV)		Up to 1 g q6h	Reliable CNS levels perioperatively	Expensive
Neuromodulatory Medications	Voltage-dependent calcium channels in CNS or PNS		Reduces opioid use and opioid-related side effects	
Gabapentin (PO)		300 mg tid		Dizziness, drowsiness, ataxia, fatigue
Pregabalin (PO)		75–100 mg q12h		Dizziness, somnolence, visual disturbances
Opioid Agonists				Constipation, nausea, pruritis, respiratory depression

(continued on next page)

Table 1
(continued)

Medication	Mechanism of Action	Dosing	Positive Features	Side Effects/Complications
Oxycodone (PO)	Mu receptor agonist	5–15 mg q3–6h		
Combined Opioid Agonist SNRIs	Mu agonist and SNRI			Caution use with other SSRIs such as SSRI antidepressants
Tramadol (PO)	Serotonin and norepinephrine reuptake inhibitor	50–100 mg q6h	Lower risk of tolerance/dependence	Flushing, dizziness, headache, drowsiness, insomnia
Tapentadol (PO)	Norepinephrine reuptake inhibitor only	50–75 mg q6h	Lower risk of tolerance/dependence, nausea, constipation	Dizziness, drowsiness, fatigue, insomnia
Glucocorticoids				
Dexamethasone (PO)		0.1 mg/kg dose preoperative or postoperative	Decrease nausea, decrease opioid use	Cardiovascular risk, CNS effects, decreased glucose tolerance
N-Methyl-ᴅ-aspartate antagonists	Modulate central sensitization of nociceptive stimulation			
Ketamine (IV)		Initial bolus 0.5 mg/kg, intraoperative 0.1 mg/kg/h, can continue same dose 48 h	Less opioid requirements postoperative	Agitation, confusion, hallucinations, muscle tremors, HTN, high abuse potential
Memantine (PO)		Start 5–10 mg bid, titrate/wk to 30 mg/d	Well tolerated	Psychosis

Abbreviations: CNS, central nervous system; HTN, hypertension; OTC, over the counter; PNS, peripheral nervous system; PO, by mouth; SNRI, selective norepinephrine reuptake inhibitor; SSRI, selective serotonin reuptake inhibitor; tid, 3 times per day.

Neuromodulatory Medications

Gabapentin and pregabalin have been proved to be useful adjuncts in perioperative pain control.[19] Although not standard, they may be helpful adjuncts in larger hallux valgus procedures, with anticipated significant postoperative pain.

Glucocorticoids

A single or double dose of systemic dexamethasone administered perioperatively has been shown to decrease narcotic consumption and improve pain control, without affecting wound healing. In a systematic review and meta-analysis of 5796 patients receiving perioperative dexamethasone across 45 studies, authors found improved pain control, decreased opioid usage, and shorter hospital stays after a single IV dose of dexamethasone 1.5 to 20.0 mg perioperatively.[20]

In a randomized controlled trial of 50 patients receiving 9 mg of dexamethasone pre-operatively and 24 hours postoperatively, patients demonstrated less oxycodone consumption (45 pills in the dexamethasone group vs 78 in the control group), decreased immediate postoperative pain scores, and decreased postoperative nausea without an increase in complications.[21]

Neuraxial anesthesia

Neuraxial anesthesia is effective in controlling postoperative pain and is a useful as an adjunct or alternative to general anesthesia to limit postoperative nausea, sedation, and delirium. However, spinal anesthesia has inherent risks, including neurologic injury and infection, which may be severe, and are not encountered in regional anesthesia. Several studies have demonstrated that popliteal nerve blocks may be preferable to spinal anesthesia, increasing patient satisfaction and pain control while decreasing the undesirable side effects seen in spinal anesthesia.

In a recent randomized, controlled trial comparing spinal anesthesia with popliteal nerve block in patients undergoing hallux valgus repair,[4] the authors recommended peripheral nerve blocks as the preferred method of anesthesia. The popliteal nerve block groups demonstrated better pain control within the first 12 hours of surgery, longer times to first postoperative analgesic, and increased pain satisfaction. The authors observed none of the anesthesia-related adverse effects seen in the spinal anesthesia group in the popliteal block group. The spinal anesthesia group showed complications of hypotension in 6.3% of patients, bradycardia in 3.3% of patients, urinary retention in 3.3% of patients, and postdural puncture headache in 10% of patients.

In a prospective trial of 40 patients comparing popliteal sciatic nerve block to spinal anesthesia, investigators[22] found patient satisfaction was slightly higher in the popliteal sciatic nerve block group, and that patient satisfaction was greater than 95% with the popliteal block. Similar to the 2016 study by Karaarslan and associates,[4] the popliteal block group did not demonstrate any of adverse anesthesia-related events seen in the spinal anesthesia group, which included hypotension (15%), bradycardia (10%), nausea/vomiting (5%), postdural puncture headache (10%), and urinary retention (20%). Although the spinal anesthesia group exhibited shorter time from anesthesia to the start of surgery and overall procedure time when compared with the popliteal nerve block group, the authors concluded that popliteal nerve blocks are the preferred modality for anesthesia in hallux valgus surgery when compared with neuraxial anesthesia.

Locoregional anesthesia includes neuraxial anesthesia (spinal, epidural), peripheral nerve blocks (sciatic, popliteal), field blocks (ankle block: post tibial, saphenous, sural, superficial and deep peroneal nerves; digital block), and wound infiltration. Regional anesthesia has increasingly expanded its role to become the preferred modality of anesthesia in patients undergoing hallux valgus surgery, owing to a variety of factors related to cost, patient outcomes, and its reduced side effects compared with regional and neuraxial anesthesia.[23,24] General anesthesia has been shown to be associated with increased cardiovascular and pulmonary risks, as well as a higher incidence of postoperative nausea, somnolence, and delirium.[25] Neuraxial anesthesia similarly carries significantly higher risks of severe, debilitating complications, including cardiac arrest and neurologic complications.[26] Furthermore, neuraxial anesthesia is associated with the additional risks of urinary retention, intraoperative hypotension and bradycardia, postdural puncture headache, which are not complications experienced with peripheral nerve block.[22] Regional anesthesia is associated with a decreased cost of care, shorter length of stay, and facilitates outpatient surgery.[27–30] With the increasing transition to ambulatory surgery, there is an increasing emphasis on the effective control of postoperative pain and a decreasing reliance on opiate medications, minimizing the use of sedation and avoiding the side effects common to general anesthesia. Studies have shown that regional anesthesia leads to reduced opioid requirements, reduced pain scores, and faster recovery times with an excellent safety profile.[6,31–34] Patients reported greater satisfaction scores after regional anesthesia when compared with general anesthesia and conventional, systemic analgesia while minimizing the traditional postoperative nausea and decreased alertness associated with general anesthetics and narcotic medication.[5,35–37]

Peripheral Nerve Blocks

Sciatic/popliteal nerve blocks

Studies assessing sciatic nerve blocks at both the hip proximally and distally at the knee have consistently demonstrated excellent pain relief with minimal complications, and as such these should be considered as a first line choice for hallux valgus surgery.[3–7] When compared with distal nerve blocks at the knee (popliteal sciatic nerve), proximal nerve blocks at the hip (sciatic and femoral nerves) have not shown any superiority in pain control.[2] However, there has been shown to be an increase in the incidence of falls and a delay in ambulation with proximal peripheral nerve blocks,[2,38] thereby increasing the appeal of peripheral blocks completed at the knee.

When compared with peripheral blockade at the ankle, popliteal sciatic nerve blocks have been shown to longer duration of anesthesia, although similar rates of patient satisfaction have been noted with each procedure.[39] In a randomized controlled trial, authors observed longer duration of analgesia with popliteal nerve block when compared with peripheral nerve blockade at the ankle (14 hours vs 11 hours), although similar rates of patient satisfaction (92% in ankle group, and 96% in popliteal group were observed.) There were no anesthesia related complications in either group.

Continuous infusion of local anesthetic with sciatic nerve blockade has been shown to increase the duration of analgesia, decrease readmissions after hallux valgus surgery, with minimal catheter-related complications.[2,6,30] Significant variations in combinations and concentrations of different local anesthetics have been described and tested in several randomized, controlled trials, and long-acting anesthetics demonstrate excellent performance, but no clear benefit has been noted of one long-acting local anesthetic over another (ie, bupivacaine, ropivacaine, and levobupivacaine).[2] Additionally the use of additives into infusions such as clonidine or fentanyl has not shown any difference or improvement in pain control, and cannot be recommended.[2]

Ankle (post tibial, saphenous, sural, superficial and deep peroneal nerves)

Single injection ankle blocks are well-established and safe techniques for forefoot surgery, supported by a large amount of evidence to be safe and effective with a high degree of patient satisfaction,[40–42] although postoperative analgesia may be shorter than with popliteal nerve blockade.[39]

Continuous postoperative field blockades with catheters have not demonstrated good success in pain control. In a level 1 randomized controlled trial,[43] the investigators did not find an improvement in postoperative pain control with postoperative continuous local infusion of anesthetic in comparison to placebo in 100 patients undergoing hallux valgus surgery (catheter placed anterior to the medial malleolus: with goal of saphenous and dorsomedial cutaneous branch of the superficial peroneal nerve field blockade).

Wound Infiltration

Infiltration with dexamethasone or lidocaine or bupivacaine has a positive effect on pain control. Neither lidocaine or dexamethasone have been proven to increase infection risk or wound complications in nondiabetic patients. It is a quick, inexpensive, and effective adjunct in the management and prevention of postoperative pain.

Liposomal bupivacaine has been of recent interest in use as an adjunct at the time of surgery, given its increased duration of action, peaking interest in potential for longer lasting pain control, and increased patient satisfaction, particularly in the immediate postoperative period. A recent prospective trial that compared patients who received liposomal bupivacaine infiltration at the cessation of forefoot surgery with those who did not demonstrated significantly decreased narcotic pill consumption on postoperative days 1 and 2. There was a trend toward lower pain scores in the immediate postoperative period, and fewer medication refills in the liposomal bupivacaine group. There were no increased complications with the infiltration group.[44]

Tourniquet insufflation

Tourniquet insufflation before the administration of an ankle block seems to provide better pain control than after the block,[45] and less pain when applied at the ankle.[46]

Choice of Anesthesia for Minimally Invasive Hallux Valgus Surgery

Minimally invasive surgery, such as percutaneous chevron or Akin osteotomies, have become increasingly common in hallux valgus surgery owing to the decreased soft tissue trauma, fewer wound complications, and significantly less postoperative pain when compared with open hallux valgus correction.[47,48] Given the decreased severity and incidence of postoperative pain with percutaneous procedures, more distal blocks at the ankle may prove an appropriate choice by the surgeon, because concerns about risk of fall and delayed ambulation seen with more proximal blocks may be obviated.[2,38] Although blocks at the ankle have demonstrated diminished pain control than popliteal blocks at the knee,[39] the increased duration of analgesia may prove to be unnecessary in less invasive procedures, and ankle blocks have already demonstrated a high degree of patient satisfaction in more invasive open hallux valgus correction.[40–42]

SUMMARY
Use of Regional Anesthesia

The use of locoregional analgesic techniques should be considered a first-line intervention. These techniques have been consistently shown to improve patient satisfaction and offer excellent pain control with minimal side effects. Regional anesthesia may be used as an additive to general or neuraxial anesthesia with positive results, or preferably as the primary form of anesthesia owing to the avoidance of the undesirable side effects of general or neuraxial anesthesia.[49,50]

Sciatic nerve blocks should be considered first line in hallux valgus surgery, although ankle blocks and wound instillation with long-acting anesthetic may show increasing utility for newer minimally invasive procedures with which the anticipation of severe postoperative pain is less. Because there has been no demonstrated superiority of sciatic nerve blocks at the hip compared with the knee, distal nerve blocks at the knee (popliteal) should be preferred, owing to the decreased risk of falls and association with earlier ambulation.[2,38]

Recommended Multimodal Pain Management Protocol

After a 2015 systematic review assessing all RCTs of pain management and patient outcomes after elective foot and ankle surgery, Wang and colleagues[2] offered the following protocol graded by level of evidence.

Preoperative

- *Oral acetaminophen plus and NSAID or COX-2 selective inhibitors* approximately 1 to 2 hours preoperatively, if no contraindications (with a Grade A recommendation)
- *Popliteal sciatic nerve block with long-acting local anesthetic*, if no contraindications, for surgical procedures associated with severe postoperative pain (Grade B recommendation).

Intraoperative

- *Dexamethasone 4 to 8 mg, IV* after induction of general anesthesia (Grade A recommendation)
- *Acetaminophen IV*, and *parenteral NSAID or COX-2 selective inhibitor*, if not administered orally preoperatively (Grade A recommendation)
- *Ankle block and/or wound infiltration with long-acting local anesthetic at the end of surgery*, if popliteal sciatic nerve block not performed preoperatively (Grade B recommendation)

Postoperative

- *Oral acetaminophen* plus
- *NSAID or COX-2 selective inhibitor*, supplemented by
- *Weak opioids* (such as tramadol) for low to moderate intensity pain, with
- *Stronger opioids* (eg, hydrocodone, oxycodone, and hydromorphone) for moderate-to-high intensity pain, administered as needed (Grade A recommendation)

Limiting Narcotic Use to Optimize Outcomes

- In a prospective study of 84 patients undergoing outpatient foot and ankle surgery under neuraxial anesthesia and a long-lasting popliteal nerve block consisting of dexamethasone and bupivacaine, authors noted an average of 22.5 narcotic pills consumed, with an upper 95% confidence interval of 27 pills at the 8 week follow-up.[34] Patients were given prescriptions for 3 days ibuprofen, deep venous thrombosis prophylaxis with aspirin, and a 30- or 60-pill narcotic prescription; under this protocol patients reported consistently low and decreasing visual analog pain scores, and at the 2 week postoperative visit only 17.5% were consuming narcotic medication, and only 2.6% were taking the narcotics 8 weeks postoperatively. These results parallel a study completed in upper extremity patients undergoing elective outpatient upper extremity surgery; after bony procedures patients required 14 pills, whereas those undergoing soft tissue procedures required only 9 pills. Furthermore, on average, patients consumed 19 pills fewer than prescribed.[51] The authors postulated that a higher requirement in foot and ankle surgery may be seen owing to the dependent position of the extremity, *and recommended a prescription benchmark of 30 narcotic pills postoperatively.*[34]

- In a 2018 retrospective review of 988 patients, Saini and colleagues[1] found patients undergoing outpatient foot an ankle surgery consumed a median of 20 pills of 5 mg oxycodone equivalent consumed, with a median prescription, this accounted to a surplus of 20 pills per patient.

DISCLOSURE

The authors have nothing to disclose.

REFERENCES

1. Saini S, McDonald EL, Shakked R, et al. Prospective evaluation of utilization patterns and prescribing guidelines of opioid consumption following orthopedic foot and ankle surgery. Foot Ankle Int 2018;39(11):1257–65.
2. Wang J, Liu GT, Mayo HG, et al. Pain management for elective foot and ankle surgery: a systematic review of randomized controlled trials. J Foot Ankle Surg 2015; 54(4):625–35.
3. Saporito A, Petri GJ, Sturini E, et al. Safety and effectiveness of bilateral continuous sciatic nerve block for bilateral orthopaedic foot surgery: a cohort study. Eur J Anaesthesiol 2014;31(11):620–5.
4. Karaarslan S, Tekgül ZT, Şimşek E, et al. Comparison between ultrasonography-guided popliteal sciatic nerve block and spinal anesthesia for hallux valgus repair. Foot Ankle Int 2016;37(1):85–9.
5. McLeod DH, Wong DH, Claridge RJ, et al. Lateral popliteal sciatic nerve block compared with subcutaneous infiltration for analgesia following foot surgery. Can J Anaesth 1994;41:673–6.
6. Ilfeld BM, Morey TE, Wang RD, et al. Continuous popliteal sciatic nerve block for postoperative pain control at home: a randomized, double-blinded, placebo controlled study. Anesthesiology 2002;97(4):959–65.
7. Samuel R, Sloan A, Patel K, et al. The efficacy of combined popliteal and ankle blocks in forefoot surgery. J Bone Joint Surg 2008;90(7):1443–6.
8. Kehlet H, Wilmore DW. Multimodal strategies to improve surgical outcome. Am J Surg 2002;183(6):630–41.
9. Kohring JM, Orgain NG. Multimodal analgesia in foot and ankle surgery. Orthop Clin North Am 2017;48(4):495–505.
10. Turan I, Assareh H, Rolf C, et al. Multi-modal-analgesia for pain management after hallux valgus surgery: a prospective randomised study on the effect of ankle block. J Orthop Surg Res 2007;2:26.
11. Murray O, Holt G, McGrory R, et al. Efficacy of outpatient bilateral simultaneous hallux valgus surgery. Orthopedics 2010;33(6):394.
12. van Boekel RLM, Warlé MC, Nielen RGC, et al. Relationship between postoperative pain and overall 30-day complications in a broad surgical population: an observational study. Ann Surg 2017. https://doi.org/10.1097/SLA.0000000000002583.
13. Oderda GM, Gan TJ, Johnson BH, et al. Effect of opioid-related adverse events on outcomes in selected surgical patients. J Pain Palliat Care Pharmacother 2013;27(1):62–70.

14. Popping DM, Zahn PK, Van Aken HK, et al. Effectiveness and safety of postoperative pain management: a survey of 18 925 consecutive patients between 1998 and 2006 (2nd revision): a database analysis of prospectively raised data. Br J Anaesth 2008;101(6):832–40.

15. Apfelbaum JL, Chen C, Mehta SS, et al. Postoperative pain experience: results from a national survey suggest postoperative pain continues to be undermanaged. Anesth Analg 2003;97(2):534–40.

16. Brattwall M, Turan I, Jakobsson J. Pain management after elective hallux valgus surgery: a prospective randomized double-blind study comparing etoricoxib and tramadol. Anesth Analg 2010;111(2):544–9.

17. Noroozi M, Doroudian MR, Sarkouhi A, et al. Synergistic effects of paracetamol and dexamethasone with lidocaine in intravenous regional anesthesia (IVRA) of upper limbs: a randomized clinical trial. Egypt J Anaesth 2016;32(1):111–5.

18. Altman RD. A rationale for combining acetaminophen and NSAIDs for mild-to-moderate pain. Clin Exp Rheumatol 2004;22(1):110–7.

19. Crisologo PA, Monson EK, Atway SA. Gabapentin as an adjunct to standard postoperative pain management protocol in lower extremity surgery. J Foot Ankle Surg 2018;57(4):781–4.

20. Waldron N, Jones C, Gan T, et al. Impact of perioperative dexamethasone on postoperative analgesia and side-effects: systematic review and meta-analysis. Br J Anaesth 2013;110(2):191–200.

21. Mattila K, Kontinen VK, Kalso E, et al. Dexamethasone decreases oxycodone consumption following osteotomy of the first metatarsal bone: a randomized controlled trial in day surgery. Acta Anaesthesiol Scand 2010;54(3):268–76.

22. Jeon HJ, Park YC, Lee JN, et al. Popliteal sciatic nerve block versus spinal anesthesia in hallux valgus surgery. Korean J Anesthesiol 2013;64(4):321–6.

23. Vadivelu N, Kai AM, Maslin B, et al. Role of regional anesthesia in foot and ankle surgery. Foot Ankle Spec 2015;8(3):212–9.

24. Provenzano DA, Viscusi ER, Adams SB Jr, et al. Safety and efficacy of the popliteal fossa nerve block when utilized for foot and ankle surgery. Foot Ankle Int 2002;23:394–9.

25. Kettner SC, Willschke H, Marhofer P. Does regional anaesthesia really improve outcome? Br J Anaesth 2011;107(Suppl 1):I90–5.

26. Auroy Y, Narchi P, Messiah A, et al. Serious complications related to regional anesthesia: results of a prospective survey in France. Anesthesiology 1997;87(3):479–86.

27. Collins L, Halwani A, Vaghadia H. Impact of a regional anesthesia analgesia program for outpatient foot surgery. Can J Anaesth 1999;46:840–5.

28. Williams BA, Kentor ML, Vogt MT, et al. Economics of nerve block pain management after anterior cruciate ligament reconstruction: potential hospital cost savings via associated postanesthesia care unit bypass and same-day discharge. Anesthesiology 2004;100:697–706.

29. Foote J, Freeman R, Morgan S, et al. Surgeon administered regional blocks for day case forefoot surgery. Foot Ankle Surg 2012;18(2):141–3.

30. Saporito A, Sturini E, Borgeat A, et al. The effect of continuous popliteal sciatic nerve block on unplanned postoperative visits and readmissions after foot surgery – a randomised, controlled study comparing day-care and inpatient management. Anaesthesia 2014;69(11):1197–205.

31. di Benedetto P, Casati A, Bertini L. Continuous subgluteus sciatic nerve block after orthopedic foot and ankle surgery: comparison of two infusion techniques. Reg Anesth Pain Med 2002;27:168–72.

32. Zaric D, Boysen K, Christiansen J, et al. Continuous popliteal sciatic nerve block for outpatient foot surgery – a randomized, controlled trial. Acta Anaesthesiol Scand 2004;48(3):337–41.

33. Kir MC, Kir G. Ankle nerve block adjuvant to general anesthesia reduces postsurgical pain and improves functional outcomes in hallux valgus surgery. Med Princ Pract 2018;27(3):236–40.

34. Gupta A, Kumar K, Roberts MM, et al. Pain management after outpatient foot and ankle surgery. Foot Ankle Int 2018;39(2):149–54.

35. Grosser DM, Herr MJ, Claridge RJ, et al. Preoperative lateral popliteal nerve block for intraoperative and postoperative pain control in elective foot and ankle surgery: a prospective analysis. Foot Ankle Int 2007;28(12):1271–5.

36. Rongstad K, Mann RA, Prieskorn D, et al. Popliteal sciatic nerve block for postoperative analgesia. Foot Ankle Int 1996;17(7):378–82.

37. Borgeat A, Ekatodramis G, Schenker CA. Postoperative nausea and vomiting in regional anesthesia: a review. Anesthesiology 2003;98(2):530–47.

38. Johnson RL, Kopp SL, Hebl JR, et al. Falls and major orthopaedic surgery with peripheral nerve blockade: a systematic review and meta-analysis. Br J Anaesth 2013;110:518–28.

39. Migues A, Slullitel G, Vescovo A, et al. Peripheral foot blockade versus popliteal fossa nerve block: a prospective randomized trial in 51 patients. J Foot Ankle Surg 2005;44: 354–7.

40. Pearce CJ, Hamilton PD. Current concepts review: regional anesthesia for foot and ankle surgery. Foot Ankle Int 2010;31(8):732–9.

41. Delgado-Martínez AD, Marchal JM. Supramalleolar ankle block anesthesia and ankle tourniquet for foot surgery. Foot Ankle 2001;22:836–8.

42. Kullenberg B, Topalis C, Resch S. Ankle nerve block—perioperative pain relief in surgery of the forefoot. Foot 2006;16:135–7.

43. Rose B, Kunasingam K, Barton T, et al. A randomized controlled trial assessing the effect of a continuous subcutaneous infusion of local anesthetic following elective surgery to the great toe. Foot Ankle Spec 2017;10(2):116–24.

44. Robbins J, Green CL, Parekh SG. Liposomal bupivacaine in forefoot surgery. Foot Ankle Int 2015;36(5):503–7.

45. Singh VK, Ridgers S, Sott AH. Ankle block in forefoot reconstruction before or after inflation of tourniquet—does timing matter? Foot Ankle Surg 2013;19(1):15–7.

46. Finsen V, Kasseth AM. Tourniquets in forefoot surgery: less pain when placed at the ankle. J Bone Joint Surg Br 1997;79(1):99–101.

47. Lee M, Walsh J, Smith MM, et al. Hallux valgus correction comparing percutaneous chevron/akin (PECA) and open scarf/akin osteotomies. Foot Ankle Int 2017;38(8): 838–46.

48. Lai MC, Rikhraj IS, Woo YL, et al. Clinical and radiological outcomes comparing percutaneous chevron-akin osteotomies vs open scarf-akin osteotomies for hallux valgus. Foot Ankle Int 2018;39(3):311–7.

49. Power I, McCormack JG, Myles PS. Regional anaesthesia and pain management. Anaesthesia 2010;65(suppl 1):38–47.

50. Stein BE, Srikumaran U, Tan EW, et al. Lower-extremity peripheral nerve blocks in the perioperative pain management of orthopaedic patients: AAOS exhibit selection. J Bone Joint Surg Am 2012;94:e167.

51. Rodgers J, Cunningham K, Fitzgerald K, et al. Opioid consumption following outpatient upper extremity surgery. J Hand Surg 2012;37(4):645–50.

Management of Hallux Valgus in Metatarsus Adductus

Sudheer C. Reddy, MD

KEYWORDS

- Metatarsus adductus • Hallux valgus • Metatarsus primus varus
- Metatarsal osteotomy • Metatarsal arthrodesis

KEY POINTS

- Metatarsus adductus is a common clinical entity that can increase the risk of developing hallux valgus and risk of recurrence following treatment.
- Multiple radiographic methods exist to evaluate for metatarsus adductus, with the Sgarlato and Engel methods most frequently used.
- Treatment must be tailored to the individual patients, accounting for the severity of the deformity and coexisting lesser toe deformities.
- Surgical treatment must take into account the low intermetatarsal 1 angle when planning the operative approach.
- Addressing all deformities, particularly in severe cases, can result in satisfactory long-term clinical outcomes.

INTRODUCTION

Metatarsus adductus is the most common congenital foot condition, with a prevalence of approximately 1 to 2 cases per 1000 births.[1,2] The deformity is characterized by adduction of the metatarsals at the level of the tarsometatarsal (TMT) articulation, often resulting in contracted medial soft tissue structures and a prominent lateral border of the foot.[1–4] Multiple causes have been proposed, including intrauterine abnormalities, osseous development, genetic predisposition, and muscular imbalance.[1,2] Although most cases of metatarsus adductus resolve by the time of skeletal maturity, persistence of the deformity has been associated with the development of hallux valgus.[4,5]

Management of concomitant hallux valgus in the setting of metatarsus adductus can be clinically challenging. The adduction of the metatarsal shafts in relation to the orientation of the tarsal bones limits the available space for correction of the

Department of Orthopaedic Surgery, Shady Grove Orthopaedics, Adventist Medical Center, George Washington University, 9601 Blackwell Road, Suite 100, Rockville, MD 20850, USA
E-mail address: sreddy8759@yahoo.com

Foot Ankle Clin N Am 25 (2020) 59–68
https://doi.org/10.1016/j.fcl.2019.10.003
1083-7515/20/© 2019 Elsevier Inc. All rights reserved.

foot.theclinics.com

deformity.[6,7] Frequently coexisting lesser toe deformities also add to the complexity of cases and the ability to achieve a successful outcome. Treatment algorithms must vary depending on the severity of each case and associated deformities with each surgical plan tailored to the individual.

PATHOGENESIS OF METATARSUS ADDUCTUS
Cause

Metatarsus adductus is often thought of a packaging abnormality in which in utero abnormalities can lead to contractures of the soft tissues and relative adduction of the metatarsals in relation to tarsal bone alignment.[1,8] It can be associated with developmental dysplasia of the hip as well as torticollis, although no significant association has been definitively determined.[9] It can be differentiated from other congenital foot conditions, such as skewfoot or talipes equinovarus, because it is an isolated forefoot deformity. Most cases are flexible, and approximately 90% resolve by maturity.[1]

Classification of metatarsus adductus is primarily clinical as defined by Bleck[3] based on the flexibility of the deformity and categorized as mild, moderate, or severe.[3,10] Mild deformities are those that can be abducted beyond midline, with midline being defined by a bisector of the heel and second web space. Moderate deformities are those that can be abducted to midline, and severe deformities are those in which the forefoot is unable to be abducted. Severe cases are often characterized by a medial soft tissue crease or fold owing to its relative rigidity.[3,10]

Relationship to Hallux Valgus

There is a strong association between the presence of metatarsus adductus and hallux valgus. Aiyer and colleagues[4] found a prevalence of approximately 30% in a series of 587 patients undergoing hallux valgus surgery. Further, it has been suggested that patients with metatarsus adductus are approximately 3.5 times more likely to develop hallux valgus.[11] There is a possibility that the contracted medial soft tissues can lead to adaptive remodeling of the metatarsals or at the Lisfranc and surrounding joints, leading to the medial metatarsals adducting more than the lateral ones.[3,5] Controversy exists as to where the apex of the deformity exists, namely whether it is in the metatarsal bases, Lisfranc articulation, or within the tarsal region, and whether it can be sensitive to the radiographic method of assessment.[5] Furthermore, there is debate about the causality of the hallux valgus. Li and colleagues[5] postulated that it is a result of a relative imbalance between the tibialis anterior and peroneals. The resultant adduction leads to greater strain on the medial capsular structures of the hallux metatarsophalangeal (MTP) joint and possible failure, allowing a hallux valgus deformity to occur.[5,12]

The concept of metatarsus adductus contributing to adolescent hallux valgus should also be considered, because there has been an association between both conditions.[8,13] The etiologic basis of juvenile hallux valgus is primarily that of metatarsus primus varus, which has also been detected in infancy.[13,14] An increase in the distal metatarsal articular angle is often noted as well. In Coughlin's[13] series on juvenile hallux valgus, moderate to severe metatarsus adductus was noted in 22% of cases. Prior investigations have also noted a linear relationship between the presence of hallux valgus and metatarsus adductus as well as an increased failure rate of surgical intervention in the setting of metatarsus adductus.[13,15,16] As the severity of metatarsus adductus increases, the space available for correction diminishes, which can lead to insufficient correction and an increased recurrence rate, particularly in juvenile patients.[8,13,15–17]

CLINICAL EVALUATION

A thorough history should be taken, particularly with respect to any evidence of congenital foot deformities, prior casting, bracing or surgical procedures (particularly osteotomies, releases, or tendon transfers), and familial history of deformities. Additional germane medical history also includes the presence of autoimmune arthropathy, neurologic conditions, and vasculopathy that could affect treatment.

The physical examination should commence with a visual assessment of the lower extremity from the knee to the foot. Hindfoot, midfoot, and forefoot alignment should be evaluated from both the anterior and posterior positions, with the assessment of any concomitant deformities that could affect treatment. The toes, particularly in the presence of lesser MTP deformities, has a windswept appearance given the valgus alignment at the articulations in relation to the adducted metatarsals (**Fig. 1**). Reducibility of the hallux valgus deformity, presence or absence of first TMT and lesser MTP instability, as well as lesser toe deformities should also be assessed. Mobility of the hallux and lesser toes should also be documented as well as the presence and location of callosities. Additional attention should be given to the vascular and neurologic status of the foot and presence or absence of braces or orthotics used.

RADIOGRAPHIC EVALUATION

Multiple methods have been proposed and used for the radiological assessment of metatarsus adductus or to evaluate hallux valgus in the context of metatarsus adductus.[4–6,11,18-22] The most frequent methods for the radiographic determination of metatarsus adductus are the Sgarlato and Engel techniques. They have shown good intraobserver and interobserver reliability across studies.[5] Modifications to the Sgarlato and Engel methods have been made over time to facilitate measurement. Values for the metatarsus adductus angle (MAA) greater than 20° are typically considered for the cutoff for metatarsus adductus.[8,11,23] Although each method is commonly used, values obtained for MAA are sensitive to the method used and tend to differ based on how the measurement is obtained.[11] It is also important to note that digital measurements are superior to goniometric ones.[24]

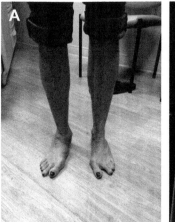 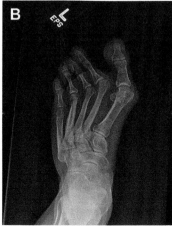

Fig. 1. (*A*) Anterior view of left foot with hallux valgus deformity in setting of metatarsus adductus. Note the windswept appearance of the hallux and lesser toes. (*B*) Anteroposterior (AP) view of foot.

The Kilmartin method is another technique designed to isolate metatarsus primus varus when evaluating hallux valgus and eliminate the influence of metatarsus adductus.[12]

Sgarlato/Modified Sgarlato Method

- On a weight-bearing anteroposterior (AP) view of the foot, a tangential line is drawn from the most distal and medial aspect of the medial cuneiform to the most proximal and medial extent of the navicular (**Fig. 2**).[4–6,18]
- A similar tangential line is drawn from the most proximal and lateral aspect of the base of the fourth TMT articulation to the most lateral aspect of the calcaneocuboid joint.
- A third line is drawn connecting the midpoints of these 2 lines.
- A perpendicular bisector is then drawn.
- An additional line is then drawn along the axis of the second metatarsal.
- The MAA is the angle subtended by the perpendicular bisector and the axis of the second metatarsal.
- The modified Sgarlato method substitutes the fifth TMT joint and has been commonly adopted for ease of visualization and reliability.[4,18,23,25]

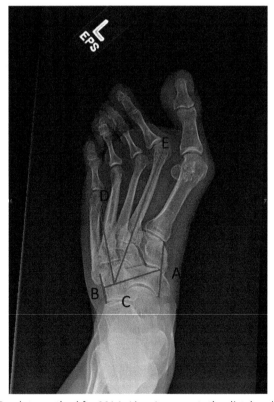

Fig. 2. Modified Sgarlato method for MAA. Line A connects the distal and medial aspects of the medial cuneiform and navicular. Line B denotes the lateral aspect of the calcaneocuboid joint and the lateral aspect of the fifth TMT articulation. Line C connects the 2 midpoints of lines A and B. Line D is the perpendicular bisector of line C. Line E is the axis of the second metatarsal shaft. The angle formed by DCE is the MAA. MAA is 32° in this image.

Domingues and Munuera[19] showed in a series of 206 AP weight-bearing radiographs from 121 patients that significant differences for the MAA were obtained depending on whether the fourth or fifth TMT articulation was used to determine the relationship of the tarsus. An average increase of 6° was noted when the fifth TMT articulation was used. Of note, in their study, men showed a slightly greater MAA of 3° relative to women.[19] As such, it is important to take into consideration the methodology used in any investigation evaluating outcomes of hallux valgus correction in metatarsus adductus.

Engel/Modified Engel Method

- Both the Engel and Modified Engel methods rely on the intermediate cuneiform to evaluate the alignment of the tarsus (**Fig. 3**).[5,6,20]
- On a weight-bearing AP view of the foot, a line is drawn along the longitudinal axis of the middle cuneiform and a second line is drawn along the axis of the second metatarsal shaft. The angle formed by the 2 lines is the MAA.[1,5,20]
- In the modified Engel method, the base of the intermediate cuneiform is used and a perpendicular bisector is drawn. The angle formed between the bisector and the axis of the second metatarsal shaft is the MAA.[1]
- The Engel method has been used owing to its ease and overall reliability. However, it depends on the axis of orientation of the middle cuneiform as representative of that of the tarsus. It tends to underestimate or negatively correlate to the severity of hallux valgus.[5]

Kilmartin Method

- Radiographic method that is designed to eliminate the effect of metatarsus adductus on quantifying the degree of hallux valgus (**Fig. 4**).[5,12]

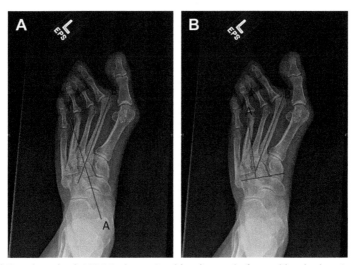

Fig. 3. (*A*) Engel method. MAA is determined by the angle formed by the longitudinal axis of the intermediate cuneiform (*line A*) and the second metatarsal (*line B*). MAA is 40°. (*B*) Modified Engel method. MAA is determined by the angle formed by a perpendicular bisector to the proximal articular surface of the middle cuneiform (*line A*) and the axis of the second metatarsal (*line B*). MAA is 28°.

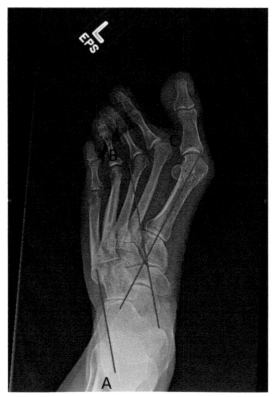

Fig. 4. Kilmartin angle. Line A represents the lateral wall of the calcaneus. Line B is a parallel line to line A. Line C represents the longitudinal axis of the first metatarsal. The angle formed between lines B and C represents the Kilmartin angle.

- On a weight-bearing AP view of the foot, a line is drawn parallel to the lateral wall of the calcaneus.
- A second line is drawn along the axis of the first metatarsal shaft.
- A third line is drawn parallel to the first line such that it intersects the longitudinal axis of the first metatarsal. The Kilmartin angle is formed by these 2 lines.

MANAGEMENT

Surgical management of hallux valgus in the setting of MAA can be difficult owing to the decrease in the intermetatarsal (IM) 1 to 2 angle. Limited space for metatarsal head and shaft translation can create a difficult task for the surgeon and potential increased risk of failure. Outcome studies include the use of both distal and proximal shaft osteotomies, TMT arthrodesis, and realignment of the lesser rays for more advanced cases. Studies are primarily limited to case series using single or multiple techniques to address the existing deformities. Aiyer and colleagues[8] recommended that management of all deformities, particularly in cases of severe metatarsus adductus, is critical in achieving a successful clinical outcome. Sharma and Aydogan[26] proposed a surgical algorithm to be used particularly in cases of severe hallux valgus with concomitant metatarsus adductus:

1. Correction of hindfoot valgus (if present) via calcaneal osteotomy
2. Hallux MTP distal soft tissue release
3. First TMT arthrodesis preparation
4. Lesser metatarsal basilar oblique rotational osteotomies to create space for first metatarsal translation, with severity of deformity dictating the number of lesser osteotomies to be performed
5. Reduction and fixation of first TMT arthrodesis to address the hallux valgus deformity
6. Fixation of the lesser metatarsal oblique basilar osteotomies
7. Distal metatarsal shortening osteotomies with lateral capsular release to address lesser MTP subluxation as needed
8. Akin osteotomy to address concurrent hallux valgus interphalangeus[26]

Although each case is unique and any surgical plan should be individually tailored to the extent of the deformities present, it is a reasonable algorithm to follow, particularly in cases of severe hallux valgus in the setting of metatarsus adductus.[26]

Distal/Proximal Shaft Osteotomies

Distal and proximal shaft osteotomies have been used particularly in the absence of first TMT instability or osteoarthritis at this articulation.[8,27] In their series of 587 patients undergoing hallux valgus surgery over an 11-year period, the prevalence of metatarsus adductus was 30%.[8] Distal osteotomy, consisting of a chevron osteotomy, was performed if the IM 1 angle was 16° or less with an approximate recurrence rate of 30%. Patients with an IM 1 angle of greater than 16° underwent a proximal shaft osteotomy, namely a scarf or Ludloff. There was an equivalent recurrence rate of 30% in the cohort undergoing proximal osteotomies. Paradoxically, there was a higher recurrence rate in patients with moderate MAA (<31°) of 80% versus those with severe deformity (MAA>31°), in which there was a recurrence rate of 20%. The investigators noted that those with severe deformity had coexistent lesser toe deformities and underwent realignment procedures (either osteotomies or TMT arthrodesis) to address them. The investigators further recommended that realignment procedures of the lesser rays be performed, particularly in patients with severe deformities, to reduce the likelihood of recurrence.[8]

In a separate cohort[27] of 154 patients undergoing hallux valgus correction, most patients underwent a distal metatarsal osteotomy and noted that the main factor affecting postoperative hallux valgus angle (HVA) was the preoperative value of HVA. Underlying metatarsus adductus was not a factor in affecting the postoperative HVA. The investigators attributed this to surgeon bias in potentially controlling for metatarsus adductus when determining a surgical plan because there was no discrete algorithm followed as in the Aiyer and colleagues[8,27] study.

Loh and colleagues,[23] in a series of 206 patients undergoing hallux valgus surgery, noted a prevalence of metatarsus adductus of 33%, with an average MAA of 24°. All patients underwent a scarf osteotomy and both patients with and without metatarsus adductus had similar radiographic and clinical outcomes. Underlying metatarsus adductus did not result in an inferior result.[23] In a cohort of 27 patients[28] undergoing hallux valgus surgery in the setting of metatarsus adductus, an isolated scarf/Akin osteotomy resulted in satisfactory radiographic outcomes at an average follow-up of 5 years. The investigators further concluded that a scarf/Akin combination osteotomy was an effective method to address hallux valgus in the setting of MAA without the need for lesser ray surgery. However, the extent of metatarsus adductus present within the cohort was mild, with a preoperative Engel angle of 21°.[28]

Arthrodesis

A Lapidus can be a useful procedure in addressing hallux valgus in the setting of metatarsus adductus, particularly in setting of first TMT osteoarthritis or in cases of hypermobility[8,26,27] (**Fig. 5**). Aiyer and colleagues[8] noted that although there was an equivalent recurrence rate of hallux valgus in the Lapidus cohort relative to those patients who underwent first metatarsal osteotomies, it would be a suitable alternative given the limited space available for translation of the first ray. Furthermore, Sharma and Aydogan[26] recommended its use when addressing severe hallux valgus in the presence of metatarsus adductus along with lesser metatarsal osteotomies. In their series of 4 patients with severe hallux valgus in association with metatarsus adductus, all patients showed hypermobility with associated dorsal subluxation at the first TMT articulation. For the 4 patients in their study, all showed notable improvements in HVA, IMA, MAA, forefoot width, and lesser MTP deviation at a mean follow-up of 25 months.[26]

Although beyond the scope of this article, a triplanar correction Lapidus arthrodesis can also address rotational deformity of the first metatarsal, often present in hallux valgus, as well as alleviate concerns regarding the limited IM space available for correction.[29,30] Pronation of the metatarsal shaft can lead to the presence of a metatarsal round sign[30] and changes in sesamoid position and the HVA, and is difficult to address through purely translational osteotomies.[29] It can further address the deformity at the center of rotation angulation, which is at the level of the TMT articulation (see **Fig. 5**). In a multicenter study involving 49 patients with hallux valgus, significant improvements were noted in HVA, IMA, tibial sesamoid position, and in the decrease in prevalence of the lateral round sign when using a triplanar Lapidus arthrodesis.[29] For moderate and severe deformities, particularly in the setting of metatarsus adductus, it can be coupled with lesser ray realignment via osteotomy or arthrodesis, as noted previously.

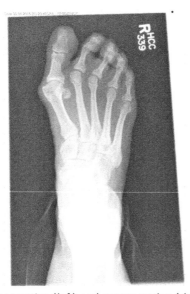
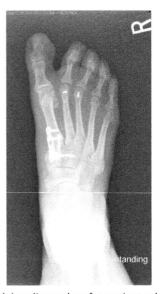

Fig. 5. Preoperative (*left*) and postoperative (*right*) radiographs of a patient who underwent a Lapidus arthrodesis and distal metatarsal shortening osteotomies to correct hallux valgus in setting of mild metatarsus adductus. MAA is 22° by the Sgarlato method. Note the residual valgus at the second and third MTP joints, which was asymptomatic.

SUMMARY

Metatarsus adductus is frequently present in patients undergoing hallux valgus correction, with an estimated prevalence of 30%. It is not only associated with the development of hallux valgus but can lead to its recurrence if not addressed. Diagnosis is primarily clinical and although radiographic methods for its evaluation vary, methods have shown good interobserver and intraobserver reliability across studies. Commonly used methods for radiographic assessment include the Sgarlato, Engel, and Kilmartin methods. Valuations for MAA differ depending on the radiological method used and are important to note when evaluating clinical outcomes of treatment of hallux valgus in the setting of metatarsus adductus. Surgical treatments also vary and outcomes are limited to case series with few comparative studies. Consistent surgical outcomes rely on the ability to account for and address not only deformities of the first ray but those of the lesser rays as well when present through a combination of osteotomies and arthrodesis.

DISCLOSURE

The author has nothing to disclose.

REFERENCES

1. Marshall N, Ward E, Williams CM. The identification and appraisal of assessment tools used to evaluate metatarsus adductus: a systematic review of their measurement properties. J Foot Ankle Res 2018;11(25):1–10.
2. Coughlin MJ, Anderson RB. Hallux valgus. In: Coughlin MJ, Saltzman CL, Anderson RB, editors. Mann's surgery of the foot and ankle. 9th edition. Philadelphia: Elsevier Saunders; 2014. p. 155–321.
3. Bleck EE. Metatarsus adductus-classification and relationship to outcomes of treatment. J Pediatr Orthop 1983;3:2–9.
4. Aiyer AA, Shariff R, Ying L, et al. Prevalence of metatarsus adductus in patients undergoing hallux valgus surgery. Foot Ankle Int 2014;35(12):1292–7.
5. Chen L, Wang C, Wang X, et al. A reappraisal of the relationship between metatarsus adductus and hallux valgus. Chin Med J (Engl) 2014;127:2067–72.
6. Dawoodi AI, Perera A. Reliability of metatarsus adductus angle and correlation with hallux valgus. Foot Ankle Surg 2012;18(3):180–6.
7. Gordillo-Fernández LM, Ortiz-Romero M, Macías JL, et al. Surgical reconstruction of the forefoot with hallux valgus associated with metatarsus adductus. J Am Podiatr Med Assoc 2016;106(4):289–93.
8. Aiyer A, Shub J, Shariff R, et al. Radiographic recurrence of deformity after hallux valgus surgery in patients with metatarsus adductus. Foot Ankle Int 2016;37(2):165–71.
9. Paton RW, Choudry Q. Neonatal foot deformities and their relationship to developmental dysplasia of the hip: an 11-year prospective, longitudinal observational study. J Bone Joint Surg Br 2009;91:655–8.
10. Dobbs MB, Beaty JH. Congenital foot deformities. In: Coughlin MJ, Saltzman CL, Anderson RB, editors. Mann's surgery of the foot and ankle. 9th edition. Philadelphia: Elsevier Saunders; 2014. p. 1831–61.
11. La Reaux RL, Lee BR. Metatarsus adductus and hallux abductovalgus: their correlation. J Foot Surg 1987;26:304–8.

12. Kilmartin TE, Flintham C. Hallux valgus surgery: a simple method for evaluating the first-second intermetatarsal angle in the presence of metatarsus adductus. J Foot Ankle Surg 2003;42:165–6.
13. Coughlin MJ. Roger A. Mann Award. Juvenile hallux valgus: etiology and treatment. Foot Ankle Int 1995;16:682–97.
14. Chell J, Dhar S. Pediatric hallux valgus. Foot Ankle Clin N Am 2014;19:235–43.
15. Banks A, Hsu Y, Mariash S, et al. Juvenile hallux abducto valgus association with metatarsus adductus. J Am Podiatr Med Assoc 1994;84:219–24.
16. Mahan K, Jacko J. Juvenile hallux valgus with compensated metatarsus adductus: a case report. J Am Podiatr Med Assoc 1991;81:525–30.
17. Pontious J, Mahan K, Carter S. Characteristics of adolescent hallux abducto valgus. A retrospective review. J Am Pod Med Assoc 1994;84:208–18.
18. Sgarlato TE. A compendium of podiatric biomechanics. San Francisco (CA): California College of Podiatric Medicine; 1971.
19. Domínguez G, Munuera PV. Metatarsus adductus angle in male and female feet: normal values with two measurement techniques. J Am Podiatr Med Assoc 2008; 98:364–9.
20. Engel E, Erlick N, Krems I. A simplified metatarsus adductus angle. J Am Podiatry Assoc 1983;73:620–8.
21. Root ML, Orien WP, Weed JH. Normal and abnormal function of the foot, vol. 2. Los Angeles (CA): Clinical Biomechanics Corp; 1977.
22. Gentili A, Mashih S, Yao L, et al. Pictorial review: foot axes and angles. Br J Radiol 1996;69:968–74.
23. Loh B, Chen JY, Yew AK, et al. Prevalence of metatarsus adductus in symptomatic hallux valgus and its influence on functional outcome. Foot Ankle Int 2015;36: 1316–21.
24. Farber DC, DeOrio JK, Steel MW. Goniometric versus computerized angle measurement in assessing hallux valgus. Foot Ankle Int 2005;26:234–8.
25. Dawoodi AIS, Perera A. Radiological assessment of metatarsus adductus. Foot Ankle Surg 2012;18:1–8.
26. Sharma J, Aydogan U. Algorithm for severe hallux valgus associated with metatarsus adductus. Foot Ankle Int 2015;36:1499–503.
27. Shibuya N, Jupiter DC, Plemmons BS, et al. Correction of hallux valgus deformity in association with underlying metatarsus adductus deformity. Foot Ankle Spec 2017;10(8):538–42.
28. Larholt J, Kilmartin TE. Rotational scarf and akin osteotomy for correction of hallux valgus associated with metatarsus adductus. Foot Ankle Int 2010;31(3):220–8.
29. Santrock RD, Smith B. Hallux valgus deformity and treatment. A three-dimensional approach: modified technique for lapidus procedure. Foot Ankle Clin N Am 2018;23:281–95.
30. Wagner P, Wagner E. Proximal rotational metatarsal osteotomy for hallux valgus (PROMO): short-term prospective case series with a novel technique and topic review. Foot Ankle Orthopaedics 2018;1–8.

Role of Coronal Plane Malalignment in Hallux Valgus Correction

Pablo Wagner, MD[a],*, Emilio Wagner, MD[b]

KEYWORDS

- Hallux valgus • PROMO • Metatarsal pronation • Osteotomy
- Deformity relapse rate

KEY POINTS

- Hallux valgus is a multiplanar deformity. It is not just a metatarsus varus–hallux valgus deformity. In most patients (90%) there is also a coronal malalignment, namely metatarsal internal rotation/pronation.
- Known hallux valgus relapse factors include incomplete postoperative hallux valgus correction, presence of metatarsus adductus, persistent postoperative abnormal distal metatarsal articular angle, and postoperative persistent pronation of the first ray.
- Postoperative persistent metatarsal pronation is a recognized independent deformity recurrence factor, so first ray pronation needs to be identified. Anteroposterior foot weight-bearing radiograph and weight-bearing foot tomography are the recommended diagnostic examinations.
- Techniques with metatarsal pronation correction capabilities include proximal rotational metatarsal osteotomy, Lapidus, dome, and proximal oblique sliding closing wedge.

INTRODUCTION

Hallux valgus disorder is a multiplanar deformity. The classic description in books of hallux valgus has for a long time been just a transverse plane deformity. Only recently has the concept that the deformity is present at multiple levels become increasingly recognized. A coronal malalignment is present in almost 90% of patients[1] to varying degrees. It consists of metatarsal pronation (external rotation) in addition to rotation of the sesamoid complex and the great toe. This coronal malalignment can be seen on radiographs, but, even during physical examination, great toe pronation can be evident.

---

[a] Universidad de Desarrollo - Clinica Alemana de Santiago, Universidad de los Andes - Hospital Militar de Santiago, Vitacura 5951, Vitacura, Santiago, Chile; [b] Universidad de Desarrollo - Clinica Alemana de Santiago, Vitacura 5951, Vitacura, Santiago, Chile
* Corresponding author.
E-mail address: Pwagnerh1@gmail.com
Twitter: @pwagnerh1 (P.W.)

Foot Ankle Clin N Am 25 (2020) 69–77
https://doi.org/10.1016/j.fcl.2019.10.009
foot.theclinics.com

IMPORTANCE AND MECHANICS

When a new factor or characteristic is described for a certain disorder, it is of importance only if it changes the patient outcomes and/or surgical results. If it does not, it just helps with a deeper understanding of the problem but has no real impact on the patient (which should be the final goal for physicians). Regarding metatarsal coronal malalignment in patients with hallux valgus, it has an impact on patients given that it affects patient outcomes and deformity relapse rate. As shown by several investigators, the recurrence rate after hallux valgus surgery ranges from 30% to 70% in the long term.[2–6] Other factors that influence hallux valgus recurrence after realignment surgery include larger preoperative hallux valgus (>40°) and intermetatarsal angles (IMAs), larger postoperative hallux valgus (>8°) and IMAs, tarsometatarsal instability, flatfoot, juvenile hallux valgus, postoperative altered distal metatarsal articular angle (DMAA), metatarsus adductus greater than 23°, postoperative sesamoid position greater than 3, and positive lateral metatarsal head round sign.[2,7–11] These factors can be summarized as the magnitude of the preoperative and postoperative IMA and hallux valgus angle, presence of metatarsus adductus, persistent postoperative abnormal DMAA, tarsometatarsal instability, and postoperative persistent pronation of the medial ray.

As stated previously, 87%[1] of patients have medial ray pronation. In patients without hallux valgus, pronation can measure up to 14°. In contrast, in patients with hallux valgus, the mean is significantly higher (22°). The pronation of the medial ray has been identified by some investigators as an important recurrence factor. Shibuya and colleagues[2] identified it as the most important relapse factor. They published a recurrence rate of 51% when the postoperative sesamoid position was greater than 4 following the Hardy and Clapham classification, and 60% if the sesamoid position was greater than 5. Similarly, Kaufmann and colleagues[8] showed the sesamoid position to be a significant relapse factor. Park and Lee[7] showed that sesamoid position can even be a relapse factor identified in immediate postoperative non–weight-bearing radiographs. The first publications that identified postoperative persistent first ray pronation as a hallux valgus relapse factor were 2 studies by Okuda and colleagues.[12,13] One focused on sesamoid incomplete postoperative reduction and the other on metatarsal bone pronation. Chen and colleagues[14] published that first ray persistent pronation was associated with inferior outcomes (American Orthopaedic Foot and Ankle Society score) and greater dissatisfaction (odds ratio = 3). Another important factor that influences postoperative functional scores is depression.[15] Katsui and colleagues[16] showed a direct relationship between an increasing (more lateral) medial sesamoid position (increasing pronation) and worsening degenerative changes at the sesamoid-metatarsal joint on computed tomography (CT). They showed too that there was a direct relationship between lateral shift of the sesamoid complex and increasing hallux valgus deformity. In contrast, Kim and colleagues[1] did not show that direct relationship.

From a biomechanical standpoint, it is not known whether pronation occurs before, after, or simultaneously with the first metatarsal varus. When the metatarsal rotates, the sesamoid complex rotates in conjunction given their mutual multiple ligamentous attachments. Because the sesamoid complex is congruent to sesamoid facets on the metatarsal and continuous with the medial capsule and deep intermetatarsal ligament, during the initial pronation the sesamoid complex rotates following the metatarsal, without dislocating from its facets. In long-standing hallux valgus, dislocation of the sesamoid complex from the metatarsal sesamoid facets can occur, given an intermetatarsal ligament and adductor tendon contracture, a loose medial capsule, and the constant lateral pull of the flexor hallucis longus tendon (FHL).[17–19] The FHL traverses between the sesamoids and inserts into the distal phalanx. If the sesamoid complex is pronated-lateralized in a patient with hallux valgus, the FHL tendon constantly pulls the great toe into valgus, progressively increasing the deformity and/or contributing to hallux valgus relapse (**Fig. 1**).

Regarding the relation between metatarsal pronation and sesamoid subluxation, Kim and Young[19] described 4 different combinations. The most common type was to have metatarsal pronation and sesamoid subluxation (61%). The second most common was to have metatarsal pronation but no sesamoid subluxation (26%) (sesamoids remained in their facets). The remaining 13% included cases without pronation but with sesamoid subluxation and cases with neither pronation nor sesamoid subluxation. Note that, when treating hallux valgus, pronation correction does not necessarily reduce sesamoids to their facets, especially if a long-standing dislocation and/or deformity is present. To reduce them, a soft tissue procedure on the metatarsosesamoid ligament and intermetatarsal ligament should be performed.

DIAGNOSIS

First ray pronation (external rotation) can be diagnosed in several ways. On physical examination, a pronated hallux is easily seen, frequently associated with a callus on the medial hallux. This is a subjective and inaccurate method, but its positive predictive value is extremely high for first ray pronation. On radiological examination, weight-bearing axial sesamoid view is a better method. It provides a good view of the sesamoid functional position relative to the metatarsal. Nevertheless, based on the authors 5 years of experience using this view, this diagnostic method has a serious flaw: it is technically very difficult to obtain and inconsistent. Given that the radiograph cassette should be perpendicular to the first metatarsal axis, it is impossible to have a standardized view, given that different degrees of deformity exist in every patient depending on the hallux valgus severity, and, therefore, multiple radiograph positions need to be considered. In addition, the foot position is uncomfortable for patients,

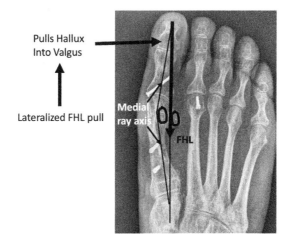

Fig. 1. Anteroposterior (AP) foot weight-bearing radiograph of a postoperative hallux valgus. As in all scarf, there was no pronation correction. The sesamoid complex is still lateralized, and the head shape is still round laterally. The FHL is lateral to the medial ray axis; therefore, a continuous lateral soft tissue pull exists on the great toe.

potentially leading to more variability and less reliability with this view. For these reasons the authors no longer recommend this view for a reliable pronation measure, classification method, or treatment decision. Kim and colleagues[1] compared simulated weight-bearing CT scans and sesamoid radiographs, and in 38% of the cases the radiograph and CT values differed. Therefore, they did not recommend the axial sesamoid view either. Another more accurate method is the weight-bearing CT (WBCT) scan. The published measurement technique takes into account the metatarsal plantar and dorsal cortices to estimate the bone rotation.[1] Even though this is a good method, the investigators recommend a different and simpler measurement technique. The angle is measured between a line through the sesamoids facets and the floor line. This technique is straightforward and fast and takes into account the functional axis of the metatarsal (sesamoids facet), and not the just the bone anatomy. Another pronation measurement method considers using the anteroposterior foot weight-bearing view. This method has been published[20] and is summarized as follows. It divides pronation in 3 stages: 10° to 20°, 20° to 30°, and greater than 30°. It is based on the metatarsal head lateral round shape. This roundness represents the metatarsal condyles that are visible laterally given the metatarsal rotation. In stage 1 (10°–20°) the lateral first metatarsal head shape is rounded, but a step from the condyle outline to the joint line can be seen (**Fig. 2**). For stage 2 (20°–30°), a continuous line from the joint line to the metatarsal condyles can be seen, but it does not form a

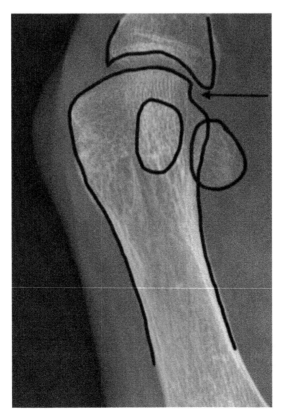

Fig. 2. AP foot weight-bearing radiograph. In stage 1 pronation (10–20°), the lateral first metatarsal head has a step from the condyle to the joint line (*arrow*).

perfectly round shape (**Fig. 3**). For stage 3, the metatarsal condyles line and the first metatarsal head form a completely round outline (**Fig. 4**). The validation of this pronation measurement method compared with weight-bearing CT scan is in process of publication. It shows substantial agreement in interobserver and intraobserver testing and a very good performance regarding diagnostic accuracy of radiographs to predict the WBCT measurement (85%).

TREATMENT OPTIONS

Surgical options that include metatarsal external rotation correction capabilities are the proximal oblique sliding closing wedge (POSCOW) osteotomy,[21] proximal metatarsal dome osteotomy,[22] Lapidus procedure,[23] and proximal rotational metatarsal osteotomy (PROMO).[20,21,24,25] These are briefly explained here.

POSCOW osteotomy is a sliding, oblique, and closing wedge osteotomy through which pronation can be corrected. The main drawback of this osteotomy is its inherent instability caused by its vertical orientation, and therefore weight-bearing protection has to be recommended for 6 weeks. The same happens with the dome osteotomy. It is a powerful osteotomy, but it is unstable given its geometry. The Lapidus procedure is another technique that has metatarsal rotation capabilities. Through the

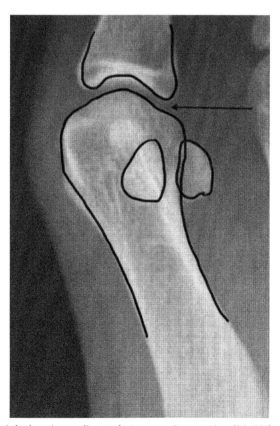

Fig. 3. AP foot weight-bearing radiograph. In stage 2 pronation (20–30°), a continuous line from the joint line to the metatarsal condyles can be seen, but it does not form a perfectly round circle (*arrow*).

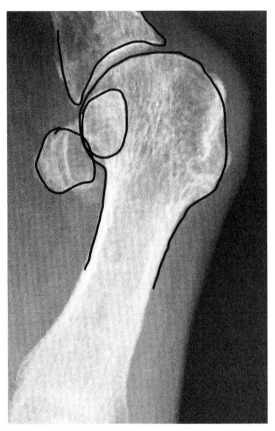

Fig. 4. AP foot weight-bearing radiograph. For stage 3, the metatarsal condyles line and the first metatarsal head are round (a *circle* can be drawn).

tarsometatarsal fusion, severe deformities can be corrected. The main drawbacks of this technique are that it is usually a healthy joint that is being fused, and that, in order to achieve fusion, the first ray is shortened (minimum, 5 mm). Restricted tarsometatarsal (TMT) motion after a Lapidus procedure can increase the plantar pressure beneath the first ray (up to 37% increase in midstance). An increase in contact pressures can also be found in the naviculocuneiform joint (27%) and fifth metatarsocuboid joint (40%).[26] Second metatarsal stress fractures may also occur because of stress increase in the second metatarsal bone after a Lapidus procedure, because stresses under the second metatarsal bone can increase up to 22% at midstance phase of gait.[27] With all Lapidus procedures, the first ray is shortened because of joint preparation, which can be further accentuated with a wedge resection. This shortening has important mechanical consequences, such as transfer metatarsalgia, lesser metatarsal plantar plate ruptures, and cosmetic concerns caused by shortening of the hallux. The overall complication rate according to Willegger and colleagues[28] is 16%. There is a 30% to 80% rate of return to activity (sports) reported in the literature.[29] For these reasons, fusing a joint that is healthy should not be taken lightly, and this should be thoroughly studied and analyzed before proceeding with it. The authors only use TMT fusion for severe cases (IMA>18°), or arthritic or unstable TMT joints.

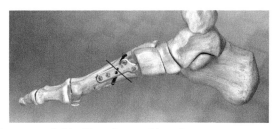

Fig. 5. A medial foot. A medial locking plate and interfragmentary screw are positioned stabilizing the PROMO osteotomy. The black oblique line represents the osteotomy.

In addition, the PROMO procedure[25] is a proximal oblique metatarsal osteotomy in which, thanks to the geometric advantage of being performed in an oblique plane, metatarsal pronation and varus can be corrected without bone resection, only through rotation (**Fig. 5**). It has a distal-dorsal to proximal plantar direction, being a stable osteotomy under weight-bearing circumstances. Taking into account the IMA and estimating the metatarsal pronation present, a precise osteotomy angle is used for each individual hallux valgus case. Weight bearing is allowed at 3 to 4 weeks postoperatively once the swelling decreases.

OUTCOMES

Clinical outcomes of techniques that correct pronation are scarce in the literature. Every hallux valgus article reports the intermetatarsal or metatarsophalangeal angular correction obtained, but not the rotational deformity correction. To our best knowledge, there are no short-term or medium-term studies published with the Lapidus procedure or POSCOW osteotomy relative to the correction of metatarsal pronation. There are some reports with the proximal crescentic osteotomy[12,13,20,25] and with the PROMO technique showing excellent and very good results. The authors' current experience with PROMO includes 60 patients with 1 year of follow-up and 25 patients with 2 years of follow-up. Adult patients with mild and moderate deformities (IMA<17°), stable TMT, and no signs of arthritis were included. Regarding complications, the authors have registered 1 (16-year-old) deformity relapse (at 3 months after surgery), 1 patient with a medium-term relapse (18 months), 1 distal segment elevation, and 1 delayed union (healed at 3 months). No infections have been seen.

SUMMARY

Metatarsal pronation correction in hallux valgus is of utmost importance if the best treatment is to be given to the patient. It has been shown in several studies how it influences the relapse rate.[2,7,8,12,13] Given the high relapse rate shown in some articles at medium to long term for operated hallux valgus (30%–70%),[2–6] some action should be taken to treat and address all the identified deformity relapse factors. The authors encourage readers to start looking at the head shape and at the sesamoids location when operating on patients with hallux valgus. We recommend assuming that any metatarsal head that appears round on its lateral aspect has a pronation deformity until the contrary is proved. If this is the case, choose the most appropriate technique in order to achieve a complete correction. If the metatarsal and sesamoids are not realigned, it is only a matter of time until the deformity reappears. The treatment goal in hallux valgus surgery should be to obtain a stable and balanced medial ray, with no skeletal malalignment or asymmetric tendon pull.

DISCLOSURE

The authors receive royalties and are consultants for Paragon 28.

REFERENCES

1. Kim Y, Kim JS, Young KW, et al. A new measure of tibial sesamoid position in hallux valgus in relation to the coronal rotation of the first metatarsal in CT scans. Foot Ankle Int 2015;36(8):944–52.
2. Shibuya N, Kyprios EM, Panchani PN, et al. Factors associated with early loss of hallux valgus correction. J Foot Ankle Surg 2018;57(2):236–40.
3. Jeuken RM, Schotanus MG, Kort NP, et al. Long-term follow-up of a randomized controlled trial comparing scarf to chevron osteotomy in hallux valgus correction. Foot Ankle Int 2016;37(7):687–95.
4. Bock P, Kluger R, Kristen KH, et al. The scarf osteotomy with minimally invasive lateral release for treatment of hallux valgus deformity: intermediate and long-term results. J Bone Joint Surg Am 2015;97(15):1238–45.
5. Deveci A, Firat A, Yilmaz S, et al. Short-term clinical and radiologic results of the scarf osteotomy: what factors contribute to recurrence? J Foot Ankle Surg 2013; 52(6):771–5.
6. Adam SP, Choung SC, Gu Y, et al. Outcomes after scarf osteotomy for treatment of adult hallux valgus deformity. Clin Orthop Relat Res 2011;469(3):854–9.
7. Park CH, Lee WC. Recurrence of hallux valgus can be predicted from immediate postoperative non-weight bearing radiographs. J Bone Joint Surg Am 2017; 99(14):1190–7.
8. Kaufmann G, Sinz S, Giesinger JM, et al. Loss of correction after chevron osteotomy for hallux valgus as a function of preoperative deformity. Foot Ankle Int 2019; 40(3):287–96.
9. Faroug R, Bagshaw O, Conway L, et al. Increased recurrence in Scarf osteotomy for mild & moderate hallux valgus with Meary's line disruption. Foot Ankle Surg 2019;25(5):608–11.
10. Bonnel F, Canovas F, Poiŕee G, et al. Evaluation of the Scarf osteotomy in hallux valgus related to distal metatarsal articular angle: a prospective study of 79 operated cases. Rev Chir Orthop Reparatrice Appar Mot 1999;85(4):381–6 [in French].
11. Kaiser P, Livingston K, Miller PE, et al. Radiographic evaluation of first metatarsal and medial cuneiform morphology in juvenile hallux valgus. Foot Ankle Int 2018; 39(10):1223–8.
12. Okuda R, Kinoshita M, Yasuda T, et al. The shape of the lateral edge of the first metatarsal head as a risk factor for recurrence of hallux valgus. J Bone Joint Surg Am 2007;89:2163–72.
13. Okuda R, Kinoshita M, Yasuda T, et al. Postoperative incomplete reduction of the sesamoids as a risk factor for recurrence of hallux valgus. J Bone Joint Surg Am 2009;91(7):1637–45.
14. Chen JY, Rikhraj K, Gatot C, et al. Tibial sesamoid position influence on functional outcome and satisfaction after hallux valgus surgery. Foot Ankle Int 2016;37(11): 1178–82.
15. Shakked R, McDonald E, Sutton R, et al. Influence of depressive symptoms on hallux valgus surgical outcomes. Foot Ankle Int 2018;39(7):795–800.
16. Katsui R, Samoto N, Taniguchi A, et al. Relationship between displacement and degenerative changes of the sesamoids in hallux valgus. Foot Ankle Int 2016; 37(12):1303–9.

17. Scranton PE Jr, Rutkowski R. Anatomic variations in the first ray: Part I. Anatomic aspects related to bunion surgery. Clin Orthop Relat Res 1980;151:244–55 (15 grados promedio de pronacion en HV ptes).
18. Saltzman CL, Aper RL, Brown TD. Anatomic determinants of first metatarso-phalangeal flexion moments in hallux valgus. Clin Orthop Relat Res 1997;339: 261–9.
19. Kim JS, Young KW. Sesamoid position in hallux valgus in relation to the coronal rotation of the first metatarsal. Foot Ankle Clin 2018;23(2):219–30.
20. Wagner P, Wagner E. Is the rotational deformity important in our decision-making process for correction of hallux valgus deformity? Foot Ankle Clin 2018;23(2): 205–17.
21. Wagner E, Ortiz C, Gould JS, et al. Proximal oblique sliding closing wedge osteotomy for hallux valgus. Foot Ankle Int 2013;34(11):1493–500.
22. Yasuda T, Okuda R, Jotoku T, et al. Proximal supination osteotomy of the first metatarsal for hallux valgus. Foot Ankle Int 2015;36(6):696–704.
23. Klemola T, Leppilahti J, Kalinainen S, et al. First tarsometatarsal joint derotational arthrodesis. a new operative technique for flexible hallux valgus without touching the first metatarsophalangeal joint. J Foot Ankle Surg 2014;53(1):22–8.
24. Wagner P, Ortiz C, Wagner E. Rotational osteotomy for hallux valgus. A new technique for primary and revision cases. Tech Foot Ankle Surg 2017;16:3–10.
25. Wagner P, Wagner E. Proximal Rotational Metatarsal Osteotomy for Hallux Valgus (PROMO): Short-term Prospective Case Series With a Novel Technique and Topic Review. Foot & Ankle Orthopaedics 2018. https://doi.org/10.1177/2473011418790071.
26. Wang Y, Li Z, Zhang M. Biomechanical study of tarsometatarsal joint fusion using finite element analysis. Med Eng Phys 2014;36:1394–400.
27. Wong DW, Zhang M, Yu J, et al. Biomechanics of first ray hypermobility: an investigation on joint force during walking using finite element analysis. Med Eng Phys 2014;36:1388–93.
28. Willegger M, Holinka J, Ristl R, et al. Correction power and complications of first tarsometatarsal joint arthrodesis for hallux valgus deformity. Int Orthop 2015;39: 467–76.
29. Fournier M, Saxena A, Maffilli N. Hallux valgus surgery in the athlete: current evidence. J Foot Ankle Surg 2019;58(4):641–3.

Evolution of Minimally Invasive Surgery in Hallux Valgus

Jorge Javier Del Vecchio, MD, MBA[a,b,c,*],
Mauricio Esteban Ghioldi, MD[a]

KEYWORDS

- Hallux valgus • Minimally invasive • Percutaneous • Evolution • Techniques

KEY POINTS

- Available data suggest that 3G represents the evolution of MIS or percutaneous surgery.
- Stable fixation of 3G osteotomy allows early full weight bearing and mobilization of the first metatarsophalangeal joint.
- Currently higher quality studies support MIS surgery. Despite this, prospective studies, larger populations, and long-term follow-up are needed to arrive at definitive conclusions on the best surgical treatment option for MIS HV correction.
- This study provides a comprehensive overview of the current literature and clearly demonstrates the variation in outcome and complication rates among procedures.
- To avoid complications, it is recommended to start an extensive training by performing related cadaveric courses, perform fellowships with orientation toward MIS surgery, or eventually attend reference centers for a suitable period.

INTRODUCTION

In the last decade, minimally invasive (MIS) or percutaneous surgery has evolved rapidly through the development of novel techniques with precise description, correct indications, and the incorporation of modifications of safe and effective techniques described in open surgery. Recently, three systematic reviews endorsed the use of MIS procedures in patients with hallux valgus (HV) deformity.[1–3] These recommendations clearly contrast with the early conclusions regarding MIS.[4–7] This is probably

[a] Foot and Ankle Section, Orthopaedics Department, Hospital Universitario - Fundación Favaloro, Solis 461, 1st Floor, Ciudad Autónoma de Buenos Aires CP 1078, Argentina; [b] Department of Kinesiology and Physiatry, Universidad Favaloro, Av. Entre Ríos 495, Ciudad Autónoma de Buenos Aires, Buenos Aires CP 1079, Argentina; [c] Minimally Invasive Foot and Ankle Society (GRECMIP-MIFAS), 2 rue Negrevergne, Merignac 33700, France
* Corresponding author. Foot and Ankle Section, Orthopaedics Department, Hospital Universitario - Fundación Favaloro, Solis 461, 1st Floor, Ciudad Autónoma de Buenos Aires CP 1078, Argentina.
E-mail address: javierdv@mac.com

Foot Ankle Clin N Am 25 (2020) 79–95
https://doi.org/10.1016/j.fcl.2019.10.010
1083-7515/20/© 2019 Elsevier Inc. All rights reserved.

caused by the quality of the published studies despite showing promising clinical results.

BASIS OF MINIMALLY INVASIVE SURGERY

There is some confusion in the terminology used to refer to MIS or percutaneous surgery. These words should refer to the skin incision/approach, not the type of osteotomy used.[8] Beside this, both of them coexist to describe usually the same procedures. This makes the comparison and analysis of published studies difficult and discourages the use of these type of surgeries. The correct term to describe these procedures should be percutaneous (made through the skin) and MIS should be reserved for procedures between percutaneous and open surgery (eg, osteosynthesis). Finally, the appropriate expression for the incisions should be portals and not approaches nor incisions. Then, one can define that percutaneous foot surgery is performed through portals through which osteotomies and bone resections are performed.

EVOLUTION OF MINIMALLY INVASIVE SURGERY

First-generation percutaneous technique was described by Isham[9] and included mainly the Reverdin-Isham procedure for the treatment of HV. Reverdin-Isham consists of an intra-articular oblique and incomplete osteotomy of the head of the first metatarsal (MT) head (**Fig. 1**). Recently, some authors published satisfactory results with the use of the Reverdin-Isham technique.[10–14] The complication rate varies between 5% and 73% when results from juvenile HV are included.[3] Actually, the main indication for this procedure is mild-to-moderate HV (**Fig. 2**).

Second-generation procedures consist of a percutaneous distal transverse osteotomy localized on the neck of the first MT and is stabilized with a medial subcutaneous K-wire. Bösch[15–23] first described the technique (**Figs. 3** and **4**) and afterward Magnan[24,25] made a modification. The Bösch complication rate ranges from 0% to 22%.[3,26] One of the main reasons why the Bösch and Magnan techniques are not used so frequently is because of their infection rate, in particular because of superficial and deep infections by the K-wire (**Table 1**). Both are indicated in mild and moderate HV.

Recently, Kaipel and colleagues[27] showed an increased risk (5% vs 30% considering trained and untrained MIS surgeons, respectively) of perioperative injury of the dorsal cutaneous branch of the deep peroneal nerve when performing a percutaneous Bösch osteotomy.

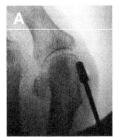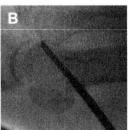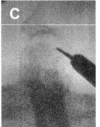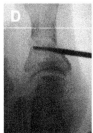

Fig. 1. Reverdin-Isham procedure. (*A*) Percutaneous bunion resection. (*B*) Reverdin-Isham osteotomy. (*C*) Lateral release. (*D*) Akin osteotomy. (*Courtesy of* Mariano de Prado, MD, PhD, Madrid, Spain.)

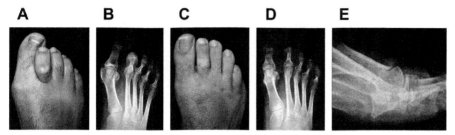

Fig. 2. (*A, B*) Mild HV deformity. (*C–E*) Final result. (*Courtesy of* Mariano de Prado, MD, PhD, Madrid, Spain.)

THIRD-GENERATION MINIMALLY INVASIVE SURGERY TECHNIQUES

Third-generation (3G) technique has been described as a modification of chevron-type osteotomy, with the addition of one or two screws to gain extra stability allowing faster rehabilitation with minor complications. In the last 10 years at least five techniques were described with promising results, although with conceptual differences among them. They are divided into extra- or intra-articular osteotomies. Some examples of those performed proximal to the joint capsule (extracapsular) are as follows:

- Minimally invasive chevron-akin (MICA) is displacement osteotomy done at the metaphysis of the first MT (extra-articular) and requires two specific screws for the stabilization of the osteotomy often associated with an akin osteotomy.[8,28–31] According to the authors, this type of fixation extends the indication of a distal

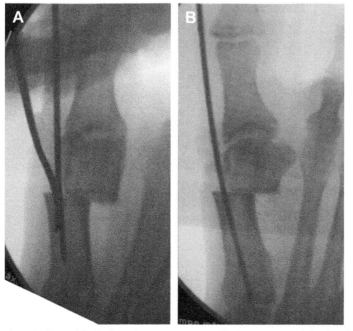

Fig. 3. Bösch technique. (*A, B*) Complete osteotomy, displacement and final stabilization. (*Courtesy of* Facundo Bilbao, MD, Buenos Aires, Argentina.)

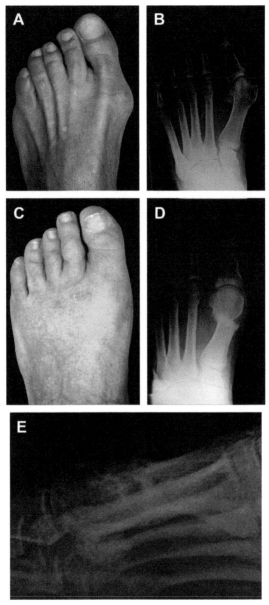

Fig. 4. (*A, B*) Moderate HV. (*C–E*) Correction achieved. (*Courtesy of* Facundo Bilbao, MD, Buenos Aires, Argentina.)

osteotomy covering severe HV cases (maximum displacement of 100%) and truly marries the perceived advantages of an extracapsular first MT osteotomy in which joint capsule is preserved with rigid internal fixation. As a result of evidenced movement of the osteotomy in some cases, the fixation technique was modified (tricortical fixation with proximal screw) to successfully avoid this problem. In 50% to 60% of cases, a percutaneous akin osteotomy of the hallux

Table 1
Bösch technique: superficial and deep surgical site infections

Author, Year	Study Type	# Feet	# SSI	%	SI	DI	Treatment
Faour-Martín et al,[16] 2013	Case series, prospective	115	2	1.7	0	2	EV ATB
Huang et al,[17] 2011	Case series, retrospective	125	11	8.8	11	0	Oral ATB
Maffulli et al,[19] 2009	Case series, retrospective	72	3	4.1	3	0	Oral ATB
Magnan et al,[24] 2005	Case series, retrospective	118	1	0.8	0	1	Oral ATB
Radwan and Mansour,[25] 2012	RCT	64	2	6.9	2	0	Oral ATB
Roth et al,[22] 1996	Comparative, retrospective	88	1	1.1	1	0	Oral ATB
Siclari & Decantis,[23] 2009	Case series, retrospective	54	1	1.8	1	0	Oral ATB
			Average	3.6			
			SD	3.1			

Abbreviations: ATB, antibiotics; DI, deep infection; EV, endovenous; RCT, randomized control trial; SD, standard deviation; SI, superficial infection; SSI, surgery site infections.
Data from Refs.[16,17,19,22–25]

proximal phalanx is also performed with percutaneous screw fixation. It showed good to excellent results, and around 90% of patients are satisfied or very satisfied with the results.[31] Compared with all the other fixation of 3G techniques, two parallels screws offer the strongest fixation particularly the proximal 4-mm screw with no risk of secondary screw displacement in comparison with the dorsal screw or the unicortical screw (**Fig. 5**). The authors mentioned that even with a 100% displacement, weight bearing with postoperative rigid shoe is possible. The main disadvantage of the MICA is the fixation with a long plantar cut and the learning curve. The difficulty of this proximal fixation is often secondary to a mistake/translation before fixation. The outcomes thus far suggest that the MICA technique may be associated with a lower risk of infection, less stiffness, and less pain. There are no osteonecrosis cases reported with MICA procedure (**Fig. 6**).

Recently, Frigg and colleagues[32] compared the range of motion and stiffness after MICA and open scarf-akin technique. The authors showed similar moderate stiffness in both groups (three cases). In MICA, extension increased by 10°, whereas it remained unchanged in scarf. Both groups showed similar improvements in American Orthopaedic Foot & Ankle Society score, pain, and subjective foot value. Radiographic evidence of correction was comparable, except for an increased shortening of the first MT by 3 mm in MICA. Wound problems included delayed healing in 10% in scarf and wound infections in 4% in MICA. The rate of recurrence and other complications were comparable, except for reoperations, which were higher in MICA (27% mainly for protruding screws) than in scarf (8% mainly for stiffness). In MICA, 14% were intraoperatively converted to open surgery. The authors observed gain in extension could be related to the increased shortening of the first MT because of the size of the burr. According to the authors, MICA showed no advantages over scarf other than a shorter scar.

- Percutaneous, extra-articular reverse-L chevron osteotomy (PERC) is also performed on the metaphysis of the first MT, and the main difference with other 3G procedures is that the osteotomy is stabilized with a dorsal-to-plantar screw (**Fig. 7**). In a case series (38 patients, 45 procedures), this technique showed an improvement of the American Orthopaedic Foot & Ankle Society score of 62.5 (30–80) preoperatively to 97.1 (75–100) postoperatively. A total of 37 patients (97%) were satisfied. At the last follow-up, there was a statistically significant decrease in the Hallux valgus angle (HVA), the intermetatarsal angle (IMA), and the proximal articular set angle. The range of movement of the first metatarsophalangeal joint improved significantly. An additional percutaneous akin osteotomy was performed in 82%, and percutaneous lateral capsular release was performed

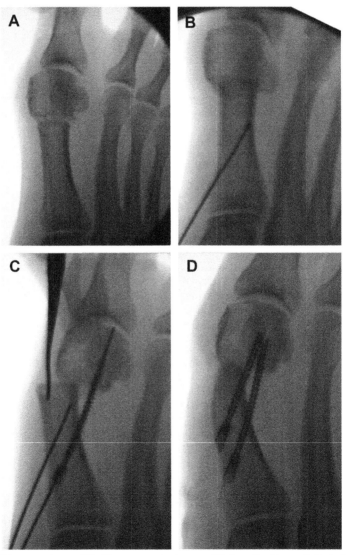

Fig. 5. MICA procedure. (*A*) Chevron osteotomy. (*B*) Localization of first K-wire. (*C*) Parallel second K-wire. (*D*) Final osteosynthesis. (*Courtesy of* Joel Vernois, MD, PhD, Paris, France.)

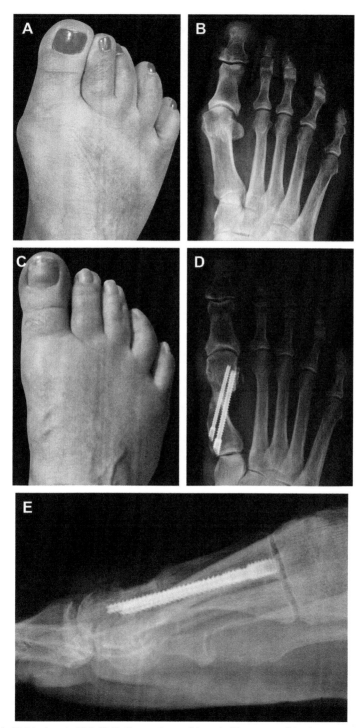

Fig. 6. (*A, B*) Moderate HV. (*C–E*) Correction achieved. (*Courtesy of* Joel Vernois, MD, PhD, Paris, France.)

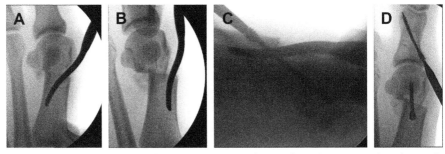

Fig. 7. (*A, B*) On completion of the osteotomy, a designed pry bar is introduced into the proximal canal via the site of the osteotomy to translate the metatarsal head in a lateral and plantar direction. (*B*) Anteroposterior view. (*C*) Lateral radioscopic view. Obliquity of the fixation and metatarsal position. (*D*) Final correction and fixation of the PERC and percutaneous akin osteotomy. (*Courtesy of* Olivier Laffenêtre, MD, Bordeaux, France.)

in 48%. According to the authors, this technique is reliable and reproducible and maintains an excellent range of movement.[33] The main differences between PERC and MICA are the type of fixation (dorsal) and the adaptability according to the displacement needed. A normal PERC needs only one screw (less than 50% of lateral shift of the first MT). In this case, the authors add a lateral screw in between 50% and 80% of displacement (modified PERC) (see **Fig. 7**). If a displacement of 80% is needed two lateral screws are used and it becomes an extra-large PERC (unpublished data) or MICA. The main advantages are: it seems to be a reliable and safe technique and easier than MICA with a shorter learning curve because of dorsal fixation (similar to open chevron). Disadvantages include less stability with only one dorsal screw, which must be performed accurately (**Fig. 8**).

- Percutaneous chevron/akin (PECA) consists of a straight transverse subcapital osteotomy. The main difference between PECA and second-generation procedures is that PECA allows dorsal/lateral or rotational correction (**Fig. 9**).[34] In addition, the dorsomedial eminence can be resected if necessary (versatility).

In a study regarding patient satisfaction, PECA showed excellent (84%) and good (16%) results when compared with open scarf. This technique showed statistically significant superiority regarding the pain level in the early postoperative phase compared with open scarf. There were no wound complications, and 24% of patients required removal of the screws because of intolerance (**Fig. 10**).[35]

- Third-generation MIS technique, described by Brogan and colleagues,[36] needs one screw and K-wire to fixate the osteotomy (**Fig. 11**). In the initial series (45 feet), there was a statistically significant improvement in all three domains of the Manchester-Oxford Foot Questionnaire, proper correction of angular values (HVA and IMA), and overall toe length decreased by only 2 mm (range, −11 to 13 mm). No cases of avascular necrosis, infection, hallux varus, nonunion, dorsal malunion of the distal fragment, metatarsalgia, and/or incidence of recurrence were shown. Other infrequent complications were described (eg, screw backout, prominent metalwork).

Brogan and colleagues[37] found no statistically significant differences when 3G MIS technique and open chevron were compared in terms of clinical and radiologic scores

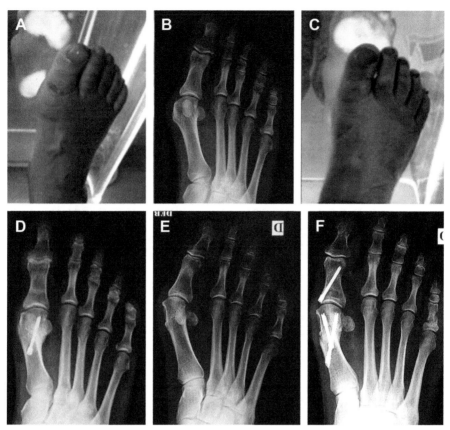

Fig. 8. PERC procedure. (*A–C*) Osteotomy displacement. (*D*) Final stabilization of PERC and akin osteotomy. (*E, F*) Extra-large PERC. (*Courtesy of* Olivier Laffenêtre, MD, Bordeaux, France.)

or complication rates. The technique proved to be a safe procedure (MIS) for symptomatic mild-to-moderate HV at midterm results.

An intra-articular technique has recently been described:

- Percutaneous, intra-articular, chevron osteotomy (PelCO): radiologic outcomes of 21 patents with moderate HV (24 feet) were evaluated.[38] This study showed a mean preoperative IMA of 12.46° (range, 11°–15°) and a postoperative of 8.13° (range, 5°–10°; standard deviation, 1.16), with an average angular correction of 4.33°. The mean preoperative HVA was 33.96° (20°–40°), and the average postoperative HVA was 8.16° (range, 3°–15°), thus obtaining an average improvement of 25.86°. No recurrence or MT shortening was observed (**Fig. 12**). According to the authors, PelCO offers theoretic advantages over other 3G procedures described because it does not need fixation with two screws (only one is enough) and/or additional K-wire, which results in less operating room time needed and complication rate and may also decrease costs. In addition, because it is done on the head of the first MT, it offers greater stability and involves fewer surgical steps (**Fig. 13**). Recently, PelCO has proven to be a safe (no nerve or tendon lesions) and

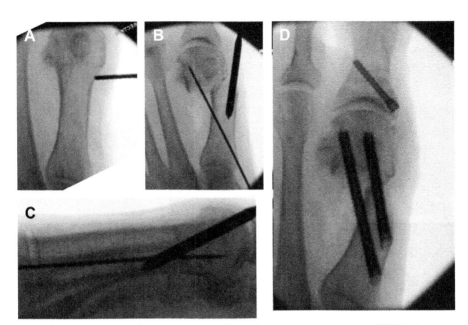

Fig. 9. (*A*) Localization of osteotomy. (*B, C*) Displacement or osteotomy. (*D*) Final antero-posterior view with two screws. (*Courtesy of* Peter Lam, MBBS(Hons), FRACS, Sydney, Australia.)

reproducible technique for a surgeon already trained in foot MIS.[39] The main indication for this technique is mild-to-moderate HV. Despite this, clinical data are needed to further validate the technique.

COMPLICATIONS

According to Malagelada and colleagues[3] the overall complication rate is 13%, showed in their systematic review (range, 0%–73%). Complications reported were comparable with the conventional open techniques, being significantly lower in centers specializing with MIS. No MIS techniques have shown superiority over others because of lack of well-designed randomized control trials and insufficient comparative case control studies.

If dorsal cheilectomy is included, the incidence of nerve injuries can reach 15%[40] or even 20%.[41] Recently, a clock method has been described.[40] This technique accurately describes the position of the dorsolateral and dorsomedial digital nerves, which were described frequently as being located between 10 o'clock and 2 o'clock.

Tendon injuries ranging from 0% to 5% have been described after percutaneous techniques. Dhukaram and colleagues[42] showed no tendon injuries in their study, including when using the MICA technique. Nevertheless, tendon lesions (up to 12.5%) seem more frequent if an akin osteotomy is performed.[43]

According to Barg and colleagues,[44] 10.6% of patients were dissatisfied and 1.5% experienced first metatarsophalangeal pain after HV surgery. The overall rate of recurrent HV was 4.9%. This issue may explain how complex it is to solve a HV deformity and its secondary complications.

To avoid complications, it is recommended to start an extensive training by performing related cadaveric courses, perform fellowships with orientation toward MIS surgery, or eventually attend reference centers for a suitable period.

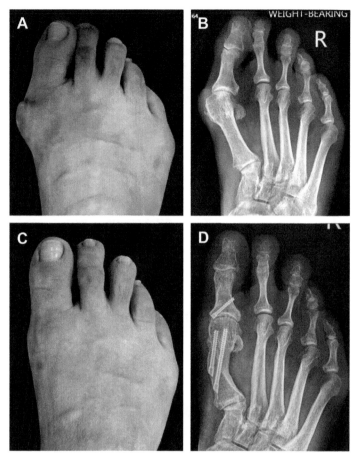

Fig. 10. (*A, B*) Moderate HV. (*C, D*) Correction achieved. (*Courtesy of* Peter Lam, MBBS(Hons), FRACS, Sydney, Australia.)

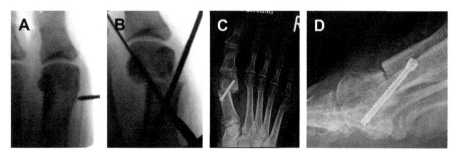

Fig. 11. Third-generation procedure. (*A, B*) Osteotomy displacement and stabilization. (*C, D*) Correction achieved. (*Courtesy of* Kit Brogan, MBBS MSc MRCS(Ed) FRCS(Tr&Orth) West Perth, Australia.)

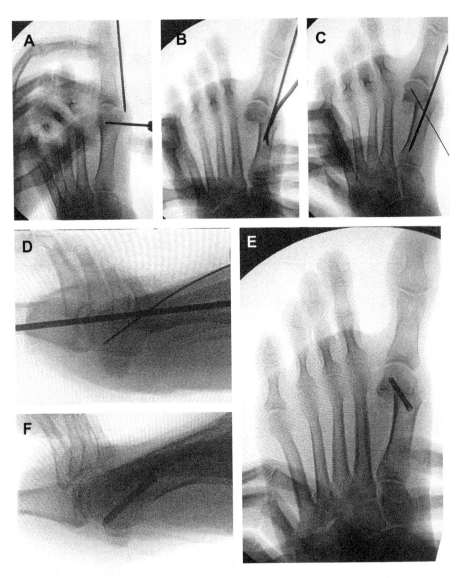

Fig. 12. PeICO procedure. (*A*) Intra-articular chevron osteotomy. (*B*) Bösch technique osteotomy displacement. (*C, D*) K-wire for osteosynthesis. (*E, F*) Final correction.

LATERAL/ADDUCTOR RELEASE

Lateral and/or adductor release is a common procedure used as a complementary technique for the correction of HV. Yet, it is not clear which structures are being sectioned during the percutaneous lateral release.[23,33,37] Further studies are needed to clearly define the correct indications (congruent vs incongruent metatarsophalangeal joint) and approaches needed (MIS vs open), among others.[45–47]

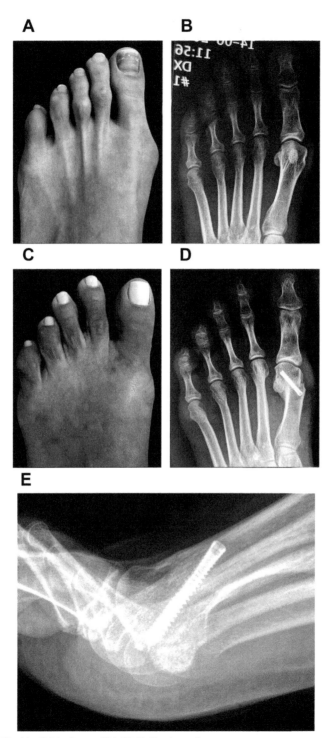

Fig. 13. PelCO. (*A*, *B*) Moderate HV. (*C–E*) Final result.

Table 2
Accepted percutaneous procedures: grade of recommendation

Accepted Procedures (Grade of Recommendation)[a]	Feasible Procedures for Possible Acceptance	Procedures Not Currently Accepted
Reverdin-Isham (B, fair)[10,13,14]	PECA[34,35]	Minimally invasive scarf
Magnan (B/C)[24,25]	PelCO[38,39]	Basal first metatarsal osteotomy
Bösch (C, poor)[16,19]	Lateral release ± adductor tendon[23,33,37]	
Third-generation chevron (C, poor)[36]		
MICA (C, poor)[30]		
Percutaneous double osteotomy (C, poor)[49]		
PERC[33]		

[a] Grades of recommendation, taken from Wright and coworkers.[48]
Data from Refs.[10,13,14,16,19,23–25,30,33–37,49]

SUMMARY

3G techniques reliably mimic the open chevron procedure with all its known virtues, but do not reproduce its disadvantages and complications. According to the results shown, 3G techniques are useful, effective, and possibly easier than open procedures. It seems that MIS surgery has an extensive learning curve, and therefore it may be difficult to imitate the results shown on already-published data. Currently, higher quality studies support MIS surgery. Despite this, prospective studies, larger populations, and long-term follow-up are needed to arrive to definitive conclusions on the best surgical treatment option for MIS HV correction. This study provides a comprehensive overview of the current literature and clearly demonstrates the variation in outcome and complication rates among techniques. Finally, based on the information provided by the latest systematic reviews and other studies we can classify the procedures into accepted, feasible procedures for possible acceptance and procedures not currently accepted (**Table 2**).

DISCLOSURE

The authors have nothing to disclose.

REFERENCES

1. Bia A, Guerra-Pinto F, Pereira BS, et al. Percutaneous osteotomies in hallux valgus: a systematic review. J Foot Ankle Surg 2018;57(1):123–30.
2. Caravelli S, Mosca M, Massimi S, et al. Percutaneous treatment of hallux valgus: what's the evidence? A systematic review. Musculoskelet Surg 2018;102(2):111–7.
3. Malagelada F, Sahirad C, Dalmau-Pastor M, et al. Minimally invasive surgery for hallux valgus: a systematic review of current surgical techniques. Int Orthop 2018;43(3):625–37.
4. Kadakia AR, Smerek JP, Myerson MS. Radiographic results after percutaneous distal metatarsal osteotomy for correction of hallux valgus deformity. Foot Ankle Int 2007;28(3):355–60.
5. Oliva F, Longo UG, Maffulli N. Minimally invasive hallux valgus correction. Orthop Clin North Am 2009;40(4):525–30, x.

6. Roukis TS. Percutaneous and minimum incision metatarsal osteotomies: a systematic review. J Foot Ankle Surg 2009;48(3):380–7.

7. Trnka HJ, Krenn S, Schuh R. Minimally invasive hallux valgus surgery: a critical review of the evidence. Int Orthop 2013;37(9):1731–5.

8. Redfern D, Perera AM. Minimally invasive osteotomies. Foot Ankle Clin N Am 2014;19:181–9.

9. Isham S. The Reverdin-Isham procedure for the correction of hallux abducto valgus. A distal metatarsal osteotomy procedure. Clin Podiatr Med Surg 1991; 8(1):81–94.

10. Bauer T, de Lavigne C, Biau D, et al. Percutaneous hallux valgus surgery: a prospective multicenter study of 189 cases. Orthop Clin North Am 2009;40(4): 505–14, ix.

11. Bauer T, Biau D, Lortat-Jacob A, et al. Percutaneous hallux valgus correction using the Reverdin-Isham osteotomy. Orthop Traumatol Surg Res 2010;96(4): 407–16.

12. Biz C, Fosser M, Dalmau-Pastor M, et al. Functional and radiographic outcomes of hallux valgus correction by mini-invasive surgery with Reverdin-Isham and Akin percutaneous osteotomies: a longitudinal prospective study with a 48-month follow-up. J Orthop Surg Res 2016;11(1):157.

13. Cervi S, Fioruzzi A, Bisogno L, et al. Percutaneous surgery of hallux valgus: risks and limitation in our experience. Acta Biomed 2014;85(suppl 2):107–12.

14. de Prado M, Ripoll PL, Vaquerob J, et al. Tratamiento quirúrgico percutáneo del hallux valgus mediante osteotomías múltiples. Rev Ortop Traumatol 2003;47: 406–16.

15. Bösch P, Wanke S, Legenstein R. Hallux valgus correction by the method of Bösch: a new technique with a seven-to-ten-year follow-up. Foot Ankle Clin 2000;5(3):485–98, v-vi.

16. Faour-Martín O, Martín-Ferrero MA, Valverde García JA, et al. Long-term results of the retrocapital metatarsal percutaneous osteotomy for hallux valgus. Int Orthop 2013;37:1799–803.

17. Huang PJ, Lin YC, Fu YC, et al. Radiographic evaluation of minimally invasive distal metatarsal osteotomy for hallux valgus. Foot Ankle Int 2011;32(5):S503–7.

18. Iannò B, Familiari F, De Gori M, et al. Midterm results and complications after minimally invasive distal metatarsal osteotomy for treatment of hallux valgus. Foot Ankle Int 2013;34(7):969–77.

19. Maffulli N, Longo UG, Oliva F, et al. Bosch osteotomy and scarf osteotomy for hallux valgus correction. Orthop Clin North Am 2009;40(4):515–24, ix-x.

20. Migues A, Campaner G, Slullitel G, et al. Minimally invasive surgery in hallux valgus and digital deformities. Orthopedics 2007;30(7):523–6.

21. Portaluri M. Hallux valgus correction by the method of Bosch: a clinical evaluation. Foot Ankle Clin 2000;5:499–511.

22. Roth A, Kohlmaier W, Tschauner C. Surgery of hallux valgus: distal metatarsal osteotomy: subcutaneous ("Bosch") versus open ("Kramer") procedures. Foot Ankle Surg 1996;2:109–17.

23. Siclari A, Decantis V. Arthroscopic lateral release and percutaneous distal osteotomy for hallux valgus: a preliminary report. Foot Ankle Int 2009;30(7):675–9.

24. Magnan B, Pezzè L, Rossi N, et al. Percutaneous distal metatarsal osteotomy for correction of hallux valgus. J Bone Joint Surg Am 2005;87(6):1191–9.

25. Radwan YA, Mansour AM. Percutaneous distal metatarsal osteotomy versus distal chevron osteotomy for correction of mild-to-moderate hallux valgus deformity. Arch Orthop Trauma Surg 2012;132(11):1539–46.

26. Giannini S, Cavallo M, Faldini C, et al. The SERI distal metatarsal osteotomy and scarf osteotomy provide similar correction of hallux valgus. Clin Orthop Relat Res 2013;471(7):2305–11.

27. Kaipel M, Reissig L, Albrecht L, et al. Risk of damaging anatomical structures during minimally invasive hallux valgus correction (Bösch technique): an anatomical study. Foot Ankle Int 2018;39(11):1355–9.

28. Jowett CRJ, Bedi HS. Preliminary results and learning curve of the minimally invasive chevron akin operation for hallux valgus. J Foot Ankle Surg 2017;56(3): 445–52.

29. Redfern D, Gill I, Harris M. Early experience with a minimally invasive modified chevron and akin osteotomy for correction of hallux valgus. J Bone Joint Surg Br 2011;93-B(Supp IV):482.

30. Vernois J, Redfern D. Percutaneous chevron: the union of classic stable fixed approach and percutaneous technique. Fub Sprunggelenk 2013;11:70–5.

31. Vernois J, Redfern DJ. Percutaneous surgery for severe hallux valgus. Foot Ankle Clin 2016;21(3):479–93.

32. Frigg A, Zaugg S, Maquieira G, et al. Stiffness and range of motion after minimally invasive chevron-akin and open scarf-akin procedures. Foot Ankle Int 2019;40(5): 515–25.

33. Lucas y, Hernandez J, Golanó P, et al. Treatment of moderate hallux valgus by percutaneous, extra-articular reverse-L chevron (PERC) osteotomy. Bone Joint J 2016;98-B(3):365–73.

34. Lam P, Lee M, Xing J, et al. Percutaneous surgery for mild to moderate hallux valgus. Foot Ankle Clin 2016;21(3):459–77.

35. Lee M, Walsh J, Smith MM, et al. Hallux valgus correction comparing percutaneous chevron/akin (PECA) and open scarf/akin osteotomies. Foot Ankle Int 2017;38(8):838–46.

36. Brogan K, Voller T, Gee C, et al. Third-generation minimally invasive correction of hallux valgus: technique and early outcomes. Int Orthop 2014;38(10):2115–21.

37. Brogan K, Lindisfarne E, Akehurst H, et al. Minimally invasive and open distal chevron osteotomy for mild to moderate hallux valgus. Foot Ankle Int 2016; 37(11):1197–204.

38. del Vecchio JJ, Ghioldi ME, Raimondi N. Osteotomía en tejadillo (chevron) con técnica mínimamente invasiva en la región distal del primer metatarsiano. Evaluación radiológica [First metatarsal Minimally invasive Chevron osteotomy. Radiologic evaluation]. Rev Asoc Argent Ortop Traumatol 2017;82(1):19–27.

39. Del Vecchio JJ, Ghioldi ME, Uzair AE, et al. Percutaneous, intra-articular, chevron osteotomy (PeICO) for the treatment of hallux valgus: a cadaveric study. Foot Ankle Int 2019;40(5):586–95.

40. Malagelada F, Dalmau-Pastor M, Fargues B, et al. Increasing the safety of minimally invasive hallux surgery: an anatomical study introducing the clock method. Foot Ankle Surg 2018;24(1):40–4.

41. Teoh KH, Haanaes EK, Alshalawi S, et al. Minimally invasive dorsal cheilectomy of the first metatarsal: a cadaveric study. Foot Ankle Int 2018;39(12):1497–501.

42. Dhukaram V, Chapman AP, Upadhyay PK. Minimally invasive forefoot surgery: a cadaveric study. Foot Ankle Int 2012;33(12):1139–44.

43. Yañez Arauz JM, Del Vecchio JJ, Codesido M, et al. Minimally invasive akin osteotomy and lateral release: anatomical structures at risk—a cadaveric study. Foot (Edinb) 2016;27:32–5.

44. Barg A, Harmer JR, Presson AP, et al. Unfavorable outcomes following surgical treatment of hallux valgus deformity: a systematic literature review. J Bone Joint Surg Am 2018;100(18):1563–73.
45. de Cesar Netto C, Roberts LE, Hudson PW, et al. The success rate of first meta-tarsophalangeal joint lateral soft tissue release through a medial transarticular approach: a cadaveric study. Foot Ankle Surg 2018 [pii:S1268-7731(18)30265-0].
46. Simons P, Klos K, Loracher C, et al. Lateral soft-tissue release through a medial incision: anatomic comparison of two techniques. Foot Ankle Surg 2015;21(2): 113–8.
47. Yammine K, Assi C. A meta-analysis of comparative clinical studies of isolated osteotomy versus osteotomy with lateral soft tissue release in treating hallux valgus. Foot Ankle Surg 2019;25(5):684–90.
48. Wright JG, Swiontkowski MF, Heckman JD. Introducing levels of evidence to the journal. J Bone Joint Surg Am 2003;85(1–3).
49. Díaz Fernández R. Treatment of moderate and severe hallux valgus by perform-ing percutaneous double osteotomy. Rev Esp Cir Ortop Traumatol 2015;59:52–8.

Current Trends in Fixation Techniques

José Antônio Veiga Sanhudo, MD, PhD[a],*, Tomás Araújo Prado Pereira, MD[b,1]

KEYWORDS

- Hallux valgus • Forefoot malalignment • Fixation • Osteotomy • Arthrodesis

KEY POINTS

- The correction of all components of a hallux valgus deformity is of paramount importance for treatment success.
- Reliable fixation is very important for maintaining surgical corrections.
- Advances in internal fixation are a major factor in improved surgical results.

INTRODUCTION

Hallux valgus is the most common deformity in the adult forefoot, and, for a long time, its correction was considered a challenge due to the high frequency of treatment failures. Any hallux valgus deformity involves varying degrees of varus of the first metatarsal, valgus of the hallux, and pronation of the first ray. The rotational component (pronation), which has been studied more intensely in recent years, is present in up to 87% of hallux valgus cases.[1] First-ray realignment osteotomies have undoubtedly been responsible for more complete corrections and lower rates of deformity recurrence. Since realignment osteotomies became established in hallux valgus treatment, better fixation methods have developed that maintain surgical corrections, accelerate consolidation, and allow earlier rehabilitation.

A complete understanding of the deformity is of utmost importance for determining the appropriate type of surgery. Choosing an ideal technique for a particular deformity involves analyzing several parameters. In the same patient, different techniques are frequently indicated for each foot. At least one surgical technique exists for each type of hallux valgus. Most of the corrective techniques can be classified as distal osteotomy (including those of the proximal phalanx and the head and neck of the first metatarsal), diaphyseal osteotomy, proximal osteotomy, metatarsocuneiform joint

[a] Foot and Ankle Department, Hospital Moinhos de Vento, Porto Alegre, Rio Grande do Sul, Brazil; [b] Foot and Ankle Department, HMV, Porto Alegre, Rio Grande do Sul, Brazil
[1] Av. Carlos Gomes 1492/1008, Porto Alegre, Rio Grande do Sul 90480-002, Brazil.
* Corresponding author. Av Praia de Belas 2124/701, Porto Alegre, Rio Grande do Sul 90110-000, Brazil.
E-mail address: josesanhudo@yahoo.com.br

Foot Ankle Clin N Am 25 (2020) 97–108
https://doi.org/10.1016/j.fcl.2019.10.006
foot.theclinics.com

arthrodesis, and metatarsophalangeal arthrodesis. Fixation techniques and implants differ for each procedure.

The main complications of hallux valgus surgery are related to the osteotomy's location, its inherent stability, the alignment obtained, and the type of fixation. This article focuses primarily on the last item.

OSTEOTOMY OF THE PROXIMAL PHALANX FOR HALLUX VALGUS

Osteotomy of the proximal phalanx, more commonly called the Akin procedure, although may be performed alone in cases of interphalangeal hallux valgus, is usually associated with a more proximal procedure, first metatarsal osteotomy or metatarsocuneiform joint arthrodesis. It is estimated that 10% of surgeons use Akin osteotomy to supplement distal osteotomy of the first metatarsal, whereas 30% use it when correcting major deformities.[2,3] The technique can add angular and rotational correction to the procedure, and the degree of additional correction depends on the size of the resected wedge. Although a single screw is the most commonly used method of fixation, crossed screws, Kirschner wires, staples, and binders are also recommended. Liszka and Gadek investigated the influence of fixation type on the results of osteotomy of the proximal phalanx in 138 patients and found no significant differences in the degree of angular correction; American Orthopaedic Foot and Ankle Society (AOFAS) score improvement; or incidence of complications between groups of patients fixed with staples, screws, or transosseous suture stabilization. These investigators concluded that the suture fixation technique is as good as the more expensive (and potentially more complicated) techniques.[4]

Complications often arise during traditional Akin technique when the saw blade reaches the lateral cortical margin and completes the osteotomy, making fixation a challenge. In the author's experience, performing an oblique osteotomy, from the proximal medial to the distal lateral, decreases the chance of this complication, making the correction less abrupt while still facilitating fixation, because it allows the screw to cross the osteotomy line almost perpendicularly (**Fig. 1**).

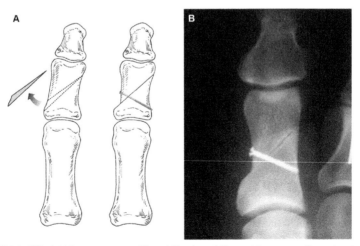

Fig. 1. (*A*) Modified Akin osteotomy. The obliquity of the cut increases the osteotomy area, smoothing the correction, allowing almost perpendicular screw fixation, and possibly speeding bone healing. (*B*) Radiograph of the phalanx after modified Akin osteotomy. (*From* Sanhudo JA. Clinical tip: modified Akin osteotomy. Foot Ankle Int. 2005; 26(10): 901-902; with permission.)

DISTAL FIRST METATARSAL OSTEOTOMIES

Distal first metatarsal osteotomies are indicated for mild deformities, but the limits of the angle used to classify the deformity as mild are highly debated among specialists. When choosing the most appropriate technique, the angulation between the first and second metatarsals, the angle between the first metatarsal and the proximal phalanx, and the distal articular angle of the metatarsal are usually taken into consideration. However, studies show low intra- and interobserver agreement regarding the measurement of these variables, and, moreover, these measurements do not take into account the thickness of the first metatarsal, foot length, or pronation of the first ray, factors that influence the magnitude of the variables and deformity correction.[5,6]

Distal chevron osteotomy is the most common procedure performed by specialists to correct mild deformities in the foot and ankle.[2] Internal fixation was not performed in the first publications on the chevron technique.[7,8] To accelerate consolidation and decrease the risk of correction loss, implants have been gaining acceptance; internal fixation is now preferred by most investigators, despite the intrinsic stability of this type of osteotomy. The most commonly used implant for distal osteotomy fixation is a noncannulated headed screw.[2]

However, Crosby and Bozarth compared the results of 3 groups of distal chevron osteotomy patients: without fixation, Herbert screw fixation, and temporary Kirschner wire fixation. No differences were observed in the results or degree of satisfaction among the patients, although the costs and surgical time were higher in the Herbert screw group than the other 2 groups.[9] Trost and colleagues[10] found no difference in distal chevron osteotomy fixation stability between fixation with a 3.5-mm cortical screw and fixation with two 1.6-mm Kirschner wires. In a retrospective study, Armstrong also found no differences between distal chevron osteotomy patients with Kirschner wire fixation or cortical screw fixation.[11]

The boldness of some investigators and the possibility of more robust internal fixations have allowed osteotomies in the distal region to achieve greater correction due to the greater displacement of the distal fragment, which not only allowed the correction of mild deformities but also contradicted the historical concept that larger deformities must be treated with proximal osteotomies.[12–15] As recommended by Sanhudo, modifying the distal chevron osteotomy angle from 60° to 30° makes the upper arm of the osteotomy reach the proximal metaphyseal region, increasing the contact area between the fragments and the procedure's stability. In fact, this modification transforms a distal osteotomy into a distally centered diaphyseal osteotomy (**Fig. 2**).[12,13] Using this modified distal chevron technique on 50 feet, Sanhudo obtained hallux valgus angle (HVA) and intermetatarsal angle (IMA) corrections of 22.70° and 10.40°, respectively, with a high degree of patient satisfaction.[13] Murawski and colleagues obtained a similar correction with a similar technique and a 60% mean lateral translation of the metatarsal head.[14] Palmanovich and Myerson[15] described the correction of major deformities using the same principle of increased translation of the distal fragment, but with transverse osteotomy and fixation with an intramedullary fixation plate (Orthohelix Mini MaxLock Extreme ISO).

PROXIMAL OSTEOTOMIES OF THE FIRST METATARSAL

Because the bone mineral density of the proximal region of the first metatarsal is less than that of the distal region, osteotomies in this region require more robust internal fixation to minimize correction losses, malunion, and/or recurrence of the deformity.

Many orthopedists perform medial opening wedge osteotomies in the region of the metatarsal base. The technique, which was described in 1960 for treating hallux

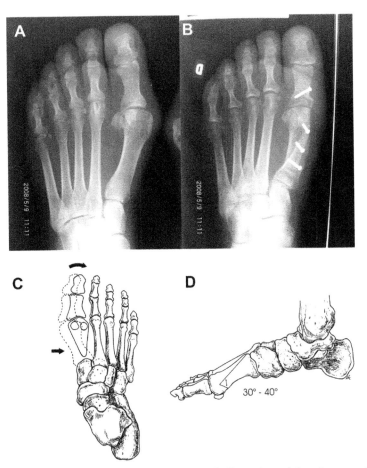

Fig. 2. (*A, B*) Radiographic examinations of severe hallux valgus deformity corrected with the modified chevron technique. The apex is distal, but the upper arm of the osteotomy reaches the proximal metaphysis, traversing the entire diaphysis. (*C, D*) The technique. ([*C,D*] *From* Sanhudo JA. Correction of moderate to severe hallux valgus deformity by a modified chevron shaft osteotomy. Foot Ankle Int. 2006; 27(8):581-5; with permission.)

valgus in adolescents, has recently gained popularity with the advent of more efficient internal fixation and, consequently, more predictable results.[16] Smith and colleagues[17] published the results of 49 metatarsal osteotomies performed to correct moderate and severe hallux valgus deformity using wedge plate fixation. The mean correction of the IMA was 7°. Complications occurred in 14 cases, including hardware irritation, nonunions, and delayed unions.

Proximal chevron osteotomy is inherently unstable because the angulation at the osteotomy site causes a medial gap, and if supination is added to the distal fragment for rotational correction, the gap becomes even wider. The long lever arm at the level of the osteotomy is also a cause for concern, because a loss of correction during the initial recovery period is not uncommon with this type of procedure. Park and colleagues[18] found a 4.6-fold higher recurrence rate in wedge plate fixation than Kirschner wire fixation (33.3% vs 9.8%). The investigators ascribed the higher failure rate of plate fixation to the fact that they were not premolded.

Bending the plate prevents some locked screws from being used and correction loss can occur when the plate is compressed close to the bone. This risk can be minimized by using premolded plates or a more recent development: customized implants.

Based on the high frequency of a rotational component in the first ray, Wagner and colleagues[19,20] developed a proximal osteotomy that can correct deformity in the coronal and rotational planes, that is, metatarsus varus and pronation of the first ray. The investigators published the results of proximal rotational metatarsal osteotomy for hallux valgus in 30 feet, with a mean prospective follow-up of 1 year. The mean IMA improved from 15.5° before the procedure to 5° at follow-up, whereas the mean HVA improved from 32.5° to 4°. Lower Extremity Functional Scale scores improved 17 points. All of the patients were satisfied and no recurrence of the deformity or other complications was observed.[21] The technique requires consulting a specially developed table to determine the angulation of the osteotomy, which is performed using specially developed guides. Fixation involves a wedge plate and lag screw, which, according to the investigators, provides great stability.

Wu and Lam used osteodesis without osteotomy to treat mild to moderate hallux valgus.[22] The procedure consisted of realigning the first and second metatarsals with double stranded # 1 PDS sutures (Ethicon Inc., Somerville, NJ, USA). Opposing cortices of the first and second metatarsal were fish-scaled with an osteotome to induce postoperative fibrous bonding ingrowth. In 110 feet treated with the technique, the investigators obtained a mean IMA decrease from 14° to 7° and a mean HVA decrease from 31° to 18°. The patients' mean AOFAS score improved from 68 points before surgery to 96 points at a mean follow-up of 12 months, but a fatigue fracture in the second metatarsal occurred in 5% of the cases. Using a similar principle, Cano-Martínez and colleagues[23] described correcting hallux valgus by realigning the first and second metatarsals with a mini TightRope. In a sample of 36 feet, the AOFAS score improved from a mean of 47.7 points before surgery to a mean of 88 points after 24 months of follow-up. The mean IMA and HVA corrections were 4.8° and 10°, respectively. As in Wu and Lam's study, stress fractures of the second metatarsal were a problem, occurring in 5.5% of the cases.

DIAPHYSEAL OSTEOTOMIES

In a recent study, Ludloff diaphyseal osteotomy was found to be the most commonly performed orthopedic procedure to correct severe deformities.[3] Because of its low intrinsic stability, the technique requires efficient internal fixation to ensure stability in the correction.

The scarf osteotomy is another popular diaphyseal osteotomy for correcting moderate to severe hallux valgus. The results of the technique are hampered by a high incidence of complications, with the most common being the collapse of the correction, called troughing. This complication occurs due to loss of cortical contact after correction, which occurs in the scarf osteotomy but not in the modified chevron osteotomy (**Fig. 3**). Murawski and colleagues[24] developed a modified scarf osteotomy to reduce this complication, which occurs in up to 35% of the cases.[25,26] The modified procedure, called rotational scarf osteotomy, aims to maintain cortical contact between the fragments after correcting the deformity. Through this technique, the investigators obtained an IMA reduction from 18° to 8°, HVA improvement from 37° to 12°, and, most importantly, without the occurrence of troughing.[24]

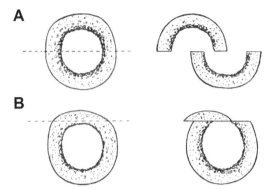

Fig. 3. An axial cut of the metatarsal after correcting the deformity, comparing classic scarf osteotomy (A) and modified chevron osteotomy (B). Note that cortical contact is lost after scarf osteotomy, a factor that predisposes to troughing.

Jung and colleagues[27] published a study demonstrating the mechanical benefit of supplemental osteotomy fixation with 2 Kirschner wires introduced longitudinally at the first metatarsal. In biomechanical tests on cadavers, the investigators observed an increase in load to failure in Ludloff and proximal crescentic metatarsal osteotomies with 2 supplementary 0.062-inch Kirschner wires compared with fixation with screws only. In the authors' experience, using a 1.5-mm Kirschner wire longitudinally in modified chevron osteotomies, especially in patients with low bone density, adds great stability to the fixation and, because of the resilience of the Kirschner wire, the alignment of the first ray is maintained even in cases that develop a fracture at the level of the diaphysis due to exaggerated effort in the postoperative period (**Fig. 4**).

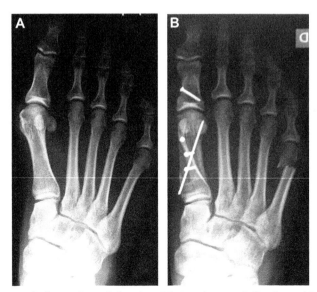

Fig. 4. (A) Severe hallux valgus deformity. (B) Supplemental fixation with longitudinal Kirschner wire adds rigidity to the hallux valgus correction, decreasing the chance of fracture in the metatarsal. Sponsel osteotomy of the fifth ray was also performed.

METATARSOPHALANGEAL ARTHRODESIS

Metatarsophalangeal joint (MTPJ) arthrodesis is an alternative treatment of severe, recurrent, or arthritic hallux valgus, especially in older and less active patients. The technique is also a great option for patients with neurologic disorders, such as cerebral palsy or stroke sequelae. The success of the procedure depends on 4 main factors: joint preparation, arthrodesis position, fixation method, and postoperative management. The ideal procedure, in turn, should be reproducible, involving a high rate of consolidation and a low incidence of complications. Several studies have found that MTPJ arthrodesis effectively corrects deformities, including the IMA, without the need for osteotomy at the base of the first metatarsal.[28–34]

Combining a dorsal plate and a compression screw has already shown greater stability than other forms of fixation for MTPJ arthrodesis.[35] Pinter and colleagues[36] compared the results of 36 patients who underwent MTPJ arthrodesis of the hallux whose fixation consisted of a dorsal plate plus a lag screw versus 63 patients who underwent the same procedure but received only a dorsal plate. The fusion rate was 89% in the dorsal plate plus lag screw group and 84% in the dorsal plate only group, which was not considered significantly different. However, the mean change in dorsiflexion angle in the immediate postoperative period versus the end of follow-up was much lower in the dorsal plate plus lag screw group (0.57° vs 6.73°). This difference was significant and demonstrated greater sagittal stability in the lag screw group.

Hunt and colleagues[37] used biomechanical testing to compare the feet of cadavers whose MTPJ was fixed with a compression screw and either a locked or an unlocked dorsal plate. The locked plate group had greater mean stiffness and demonstrated less plantar gapping during fatigue endurance testing. No significant difference in load to failure was observed between the 2 groups. The same investigators observed higher nonunion rates (23%) in 73 patients who underwent MTPJ arthrodesis with a precontoured locked titanium plate than in 107 patients who underwent the same procedure with a nonlocked stainless steel plate (11% nonunion rate), possibly due to exaggerated stiffness from the wedge implant and the lack of contact or compression at the bone interface.[38] Studies have hypothesized that the rigidity provided by wedge plate fixations suppresses interfragmentary mobility at one level, which impairs consolidation.[39,40] This scenario is even more likely in cases of wedge plate fixation where compression between the fragments and/or bone contact was insufficient.

In these investigators' experience, for patients with severe hallux valgus with or without arthrodesis, MTPJ arthrodesis fixed with cerclage or crossed Kirschner wires has presented high levels of radiographic consolidation and patient satisfaction. In 23 patients (29 feet) who underwent the procedure, the fusion rate was 100%. After an average follow-up of 35 months, the AOFAS score improved from a mean of 27.3 points before the procedure to 77.3 points at follow-up, showing an improvement of 50 points. A secret to the procedure in such cases is preserving the integrity of the adductor tendon, because the resilience of the hallux valgus deformity associated with intramedullary fixation with Kirschner wires and the action of the adductor tendon promote compression at the level of the arthrodesis and the approximation of the first and second metatarsal, correcting the IMA. The technique's greatest disadvantage in this group of patients was the high rate of reintervention to remove the implants. Although no nonunion occurred, a second procedure was required in 65% of cases due to hardware irritation. Despite presenting low stability indexes in biomechanical studies, MTPJ arthrodesis with Kirschner wires might present a high consolidation rate due to the benefits of micromobility at the arthrodesis, provided that the construction is associated with an adequate area of bone contact (**Fig. 5**).[35]

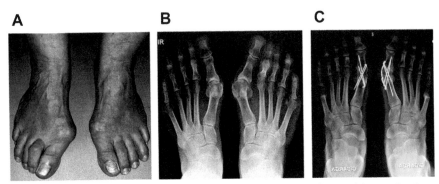

Fig. 5. (*A*) Clinical aspect of severe hallux valgus deformity. (*B*) Radiographic examination of the deformity. (*C*) Correction of severe hallux valgus deformity through MTPJ arthrodesis fixed through crossed Kirschner wires with and without cerclage. Note the intermetatarsal angle correction.

METATARSOCUNEIFORM JOINT ARTHRODESIS

Since Lapidus first described the procedure in 1934, metatarsocuneiform joint arthrodesis in the first and second rays to correct hallux valgus has undergone certain modifications, and today many investigators perform the procedure by fixing only the first ray.[41] The procedure is indicated in cases of metatarsocuneiform joint instability, which is often difficult to prove clinically or through imaging tests. Coughlin and Grebing demonstrated that the degree of mobility of the first ray is altered by the position of the ankle during the clinical examination.[42] An increased inclination angle of the metatarsocuneiform joint in radiographs has been associated with instability, but this finding is influenced by the angle of the beam during the examination and thus cannot be an isolated determinant. Doty and colleagues[43] observed that the median inclination of the metatarsocuneiform joint in the first ray was 15.8° in 10° anteroposterior radiographs, whereas it was 2.6° in 20° anteroposterior radiographs.

Many modifications of the original Lapidus technique have been described, such as the inclusion or not of the second ray in the arthrodesis and different types of fixation. Recently, traditional screw fixation has been replaced with special locking plates, as they show superior stability to screw fixation alone.[44,45] Fixing the plate on the tension side of the arthrodesis, that is, the plantar region, has biomechanical advantages over fixation in the medial region or dorsomedial, although there is concern that it could interfere with the anterior tibial and peroneal longus tendon insertions, because both occur in this region. Klos and colleagues[46] demonstrated in a cadaver study that plates fixed in the plantar region are stiffer and have better load to failure than plates placed in the medial dorsal region. These results are supported by clinical studies demonstrating low rates of nonunion in patients who underwent metatarsocuneiform joint arthrodesis with plantar plate fixation.[47] The main drawback of placing the plate in this region is interference with the peroneus longus and anterior tibial tendon insertions, which could explain the high reintervention rate to remove the hardware.[48] Anterior tibial tendon rupture due to this technique has been previously described.[47]

However, Plaass and colleagues[49] demonstrated in a cadaver study that there is a "safe zone" in which plantar placed plates in the metatarsocuneiform joint do not interfere with the anterior tibia or the long fibular tendon insertions.

To avoid irritation of local tissue and preserve the periosteum, an intramedullary fixation technique was developed for first-ray metatarsocuneiform joint fixation. Roth and colleagues,[50] in a biomechanical study performed on cadavers, showed that fixation with a plantar plate plus a compression screw provided a stronger and stiffer construct than fixation with an intramedullary device plus a compression screw.

Burchard and colleagues[51] compared first-ray metatarsocuneiform joint fixation in synthetic bones using a dorsal locking plate, a plantar locking plate, and fixation with an intramedullary device. Although the intramedullary device had the highest initial compression force, fixation with a plantar plate produced higher stiffness than the other forms.

Attention has also been given to rotational correction of the first ray during metatarsocuneiform joint arthrodesis. Klemola and colleagues[52] demonstrated that correcting varus and pronation of the first metatarsal can correct the entire deformity without touching the MTPJ. According to these investigators, rotational correction realigns the head of the first metatarsal and the sesamoids, bringing the relationship between the structures to a more horizontal and stable position, possibly decreasing the chance that the deformity will recur.

PERCUTANEOUS TECHNIQUES

With the introduction of internal fixation in osteotomies, procedures performed with burs have gained popularity with a greater number of practitioners, given that better results were obtained. In a recently published systematic review, the Reverdin-Isham procedure was found to have less potential for valgus hallux angle correction than a Chevron-Akin osteotomy, which is also performed percutaneously. The Reverdin-Isham procedure was also found to be less able to correct the IMA than the technique that uses the Endolog device, a curved titanium endomedullary nail that serves to push the metatarsal head laterally after a percutaneous osteotomy.[53] The development of cannulated screws with beveled heads for fixing percutaneous osteotomies has facilitated the procedures, reducing the chance of postoperative correction loss and allowing for accelerated rehabilitation.[54]

THREE-DIMENSIONAL PRINTING TECHNOLOGY

The advantages of precontoured implants for adjusting fixation and reducing surgery time, coupled with the emergence of 3-dimensional printing technology, has led to customized implants to match an individual's anatomy. Although not yet widely used, customized printed implants have already proved useful in syndromic patients and those with highly compromised bone structure. As this technology advances, large-scale production of custom implants in stainless steel, titanium, nitinol, ceramics, etc. will drive costs less than current levels, and the possibility of producing sterile implants in the operating room could completely change current material supply logistics.[55,56]

DISCLOSURE

The authors have nothing to disclose.

REFERENCES

1. Kim Y, Kim JS, Young KW, et al. A new measure of tibial sesamoid position in hallux valgus in relation to the coronal rotation of the first metatarsal in CT scans. FootAnkle Int 2015;36:944–52.

2. Pinney S, Song K, Chou L. Surgical treatment of mild hallux valgus deformity: the state of practice among academic foot and ankle surgeons. FootAnkle Int 2006; 27:970–3.

3. Pinney SJ, Song KR, Chou LB. Surgical treatment of severe hallux valgus: the state of practice among academic foot and ankle surgeons. FootAnkle Int 2006;27:1024–9.

4. Liszka H, Gadek A. Comparison of the type of fixation of akin osteotomy. FootAnkle Int 2018. https://doi.org/10.1177/1071100718816052.

5. Sanhudo JA, Gomes JE, Rabello MC, et al. Interobserver and intraobserver reproducibility of hallux valgus angular measurements and the study of a linear measurement. FootAnkle Spec 2012;5:374–7.

6. Schneider W, Knahr K. Metatarsophalangeal and inter-metatarsal angle: different values and interpretation of postoperative results dependent on the technique of measurement. FootAnkle Int 1998;19:532–6.

7. Austin DW, Leventen EO. Scientific exhibit of V-osteotomy of the fist metatarsal head. Chicago: American Academy of Orthopedic Surgery; 1968.

8. Austin DW, Leventen EO. A new osteotomy for hallux valgus: a horizontally directed "V" displacement osteotomy of the metatarsal head for hallux valgus and primus varus. Clin Orthop Relat Res 1981;157:25–30.

9. Crosby LA, Bozarth GR. Fixation comparison for chevron osteotomies. FootAnkle Int 1998;19:41–3.

10. Trost M, Bredow J, Boese CK, et al. Biomechanical comparison of fixation with a single screw versus two kirschner wires in distal chevron osteotomies of the first metatarsal: a cadaver study. J FootAnkle Surg 2018;57:95–9.

11. Armstrong DG, Pupp GR, Harkless LB. Our fixation with fixation: are screws clinically superior to external wires in distal first metatarsal osteotomies? J FootAnkle Surg 1997;36:353–5.

12. Sanhudo JA. Extending the indications for distal chevron osteotomy. FootAnkle Int 2000;21:522–3.

13. Sanhudo JA. Correction of moderate to severe hallux valgus deformity by a modified chevron shaft osteotomy. FootAnkle Int 2006;27:581–5.

14. Murawski DE, Beskin JL. Increased displacement maximizes the utility of the distal chevron osteotomy for hallux valgus deformity correction. FootAnkle Int 2008;29:155–63.

15. Palmonovich E, Myerson MS. Correction of moderate and severe hallux valgus deformity with a distal metatarsal osteotomy using an intramedullary plate. FootAnkle Clin 2014;19:191–201.

16. Simmonds FA, Menelaus MB. Hallux valgus in adolescents. JBoneJoint Surg 1960;42B:761–8.

17. Smith WB, Hyer CF, DeCarbo WT, et al. Opening wedge osteotomies for correction of hallux valgus. A review of wedge plate fixation. FootAnkle Spec 2009;2: 277–82.

18. Park CH, Ahn JY, Kim YM, et al. Plate fixation for proximal chevron osteotomy has greater risk for hallux valgus recurrence than Kirschner wire fixation. Int Orthop 2013;37:1085–92.

19. Wagner E, Wagner P, Ortiz C. Rotational osteotomy for hallux valgus. A new technique for primary and revision cases. Tech FootAnkle Surg 2017;16:3–10.

20. Wagner E, Wagner P. Is rotational deformity important in our decision-making process for correction of hallux valgus deformity? FootAnkle Clin 2018;23:205–17.

21. Wagner E, Wagner P. Proximal rotational metatrsalostoeotmy for hallux valgus (promo): short-term prospective case series with a novel technique and topic review. FootAnkle Orthop 2018;1–8. https://doi.org/10.1177/2473011418790071.

22. Wu DY, Lam KF. Osteodesis for hallux valgus correction: is it effective? Clin Orthop Relat Res 2015;473:328–36.

23. Cano-Martínez JA, Picazo-Marín F, Bento-Gerard J, et al. Tratamiento del Hallux valgus moderado con sistema mini TightRope®: técnica modificada. Rev EspCirOrtop Traumatol 2011;55:358–68.

24. Murawski CD, Egan CJ, Kennedy JG. A rotational scarf osteotomy decreases troughing when treating hallux valgus. Clin Orthop Relat Res 2011;469:847–53.

25. Hammel E, Abi Chala ML, Wagner T. Complications of first ray osteotomies: a consecutive series of 475 feet with first metatarsal scarf osteotomy and first phalanx osteotomy. Rev Chir Orthop ReparatriceAppar Mot 2007;93:710–9.

26. Coetzee JC. Scarf osteotomy for hallux valgus repair: the dark side. FootAnkle Int 2003;24:29–33.

27. Jung H-G, Guyton GP, Parks BG, et al. Supplementary axial Kirschner wire fixation for crescentic and Ludloff proximal metatarsal osteotomies: a biomechanical study. FootAnkle Int 2005;26:620–6.

28. Coughlin MJ, Grebing BR, Jones CP. Arthrodesis of the first metatarsophalangeal joint for idiopathic hallux valgus: intermediate results. FootAnkle Int 2005;26: 783–92.

29. Cronin JJ, Limbers JP, Kutty S, et al. Intermetatarsal angle after metatarsophalangeal joint arthrodesis for hallux valgus. FootAnkle Int 2006;27:104–9.

30. Pydah KVS, Toh EM, Sirikonda SP, et al. Intermetatarsal angular change following fusion of the first metatarsophalangeal joint. FootAnkle Int 2009;30:415–8.

31. Dayton P, Feilmeier M, Hunziker B, et al. Reduction of the intermetatarsal angle after first metatarsal phalangeal joint arthrodesis: a systematic review. J FootAnkle Surg 2014;53:620–3.

32. Von Salis-Soglio GF, Thomas W. Arthrodesis of the metatarsophalangeal joint of the great toe. Arch Orthop Trauma Surg 1979;95:7–12.

33. Humbert JL, Bourbonnièri C, Laurin CA. Metatarsophalangeal fusion for hallux valgus: indications and effect on the first metatarsal ray. Can Med Assoc J 1979;120:937–41.

34. McKean RM, Bergin PF, Watson G, et al. Radiographic evaluation of intermetatarsal angle correction following first MTP joint arthrodesis for severe hallux valgus. FootAnkle Int 2016;37:1183–6.

35. Politi J, Hayes J, Njus G, et al. First metatarsal-phalangeal joint arthrodesis: a biomechanical assessment of stability. FootAnkle Int 2003;24:332–7.

36. Pinter Z, Hudson P, Cone B, et al. Radiographic evaluation of the first MTP joint arthrodesis for severe hallux valgus: does the introduction of a lag screw improve union rates and correction of the intermetatarsal angle? FootAnkle Int 2017; 33:20–4.

37. Hunt KJ, Barr CR, Lindsey DP, et al. Locked versus nonlocked plate fixation for first metatarsophalangeal arthrodesis: a biomechanical investigation. FootAnkle Int 2012;33:984–90.

38. Hunt KJ, Ellington JK, Anderson RB, et al. Locked versus nonlocked plate fixation for hallux MTP arthrodesis. FootAnkle Int 2011;32:704–9.

39. Bottlang M, Doornink J, Lujan TJ. Effects of construct stiffness on healing of fractures stabilized with locking plates. JBoneJoint Surg Am 2010;92:12–22.

40. Gardner MJ, Nork SE, Huber P, et al. Stiffness modulation of locking plate constructs using near cortical slotted holes: a preliminary study. J Orthop Trauma 2009;23:281–7.

41. Lapidus PW. The operative correction of the metatarsus varus primus in hallux valgus. Surg Gynecol Obstet 1934;58:183–91.

42. Coughlin MJ, Grebing BR. The effect of ankle position on the exam for first ray mobility. FootAnkle Int 2004;25:467–75.

43. Doty JF, Coughlin MJ, Hirose C, et al. First metatarsocuneiform joint mobility: radiographic, anatomic, and clinical characteristics of the articular surface. FootAnkle Int 2014;35:504–11.

44. Klos K, Gueorguiev B, Mückley T, et al. Stability of medial locking plate and compression screw versus two crossed screws for lapidus arthrodesis. FootAnkle Int 2010;31:158–63.

45. DeVries JG, Granata JD, Hyer CF. Fixation of first tarsometatarsal arthrodesis: a retrospective comparative cohort of two techniques. FootAnkle Int 2011;32: 158–62.

46. Klos K, Simons P, Hajduk A, et al. Plantar versus dorsomedial locked plating for Lapidus arthrodesis: a biomechanical comparison. FootAnkle Int 2011;32:1081–5.

47. Klos K, Wilde CH, Lange A, et al. Modified Lapidus arthrodesis with plantar plate and compression screw for treatment of hallux valgus with hypermobility of the first ray: a preliminary report. FootAnkle Surg 2013;19:234–44.

48. Cottom JM, Vora AM. Fixation of Lapidus arthrodesis with a plantar interfragmentary screw and medial locking plate: a report of 88 cases. J FootAnkle Surg 2013; 52:465–9.

49. Plaass C, Claassen L, Daniilidis K. Placement of plantar plates for lapidus arthrodesis: anatomical considerations. FootAnkle Int 2015;37:427–32.

50. Roth KE, Peters J, Schmidtmann I, et al. Intraosseous fixation compared to plantar plate fixation for first metatarsocuneiform arthrodesis: a cadaveric biomechanical analysis. FootAnkle Int 2014;35:1209–16.

51. Burchard R, Massa R, Soos C, et al. Biomechanics of common fixations devices for first tarsometatarsal joint fusion - a comparative study with synthetic bones. J Orthop Surg Res 2018;13:176.

52. Klemola T, Leppilahti J, Kalinainen S, et al. First tarsometatarsal joint derotational arthrodesis - a new operative technique for flexible hallux valgus without touching the first metatarsophalangeal joint. J FootAnkle Surg 2014;53:22–8.

53. Biz C, Corradin M, Petretta I, et al. Endolog technique for correction of hallux valgus: a prospective study of 30 patients with 4-year follow-up. J Orthop Surg Res 2015;10:102.

54. Malagelada F, Sahirad C, Dalmau-Pastor M, et al. Minimally invasive surgery for hallux valgus: a systematic review of current surgical techniques. Int Orthop 2019;43:625–37.

55. Cai H. Application of 3D printing in orthopedics: status quo and opportunities in China. Ann Transl Med 2015;3S12. https://doi.org/10.3978/j.issn.2305-5839. 2015.01.38.

56. Eltorai AEM, Nguyen E, Daniels AH. Three-dimensional printing in orthopedic surgery. Orthopedics 2015;38:684–7.

Evolution of Thinking of the Lapidus Procedure and Fixation

Shuyuan Li, MD, PhD*, Mark S. Myerson, MD

KEYWORDS

- Lapidus procedure • Modified Lapidus procedure • Fixation
- First tarsometatarsal joint instability • First tarsometatarsal joint arthrodesis
- Hallux valgus

KEY POINTS

- The Lapidus procedures have been widely used in treating many forefoot and midfoot deformities associated with first tarsometatarsal joint dysfunction, including primary hallux valgus, recurrent hallux valgus, metatarsal adductus, lesser metatarsalgia, and midfoot arthritis, because the Lapidus procedures have the ability to restore the first ray alignment in 3 dimensions.
- Choosing between a traditional and a modified Lapidus procedure is based on whether the sagittal or the transverse plane motion between the first and second rays is acceptable or not. Too much mobility in either plane can lead to recurrent deformity, and it is suggested to start with a modified Lapidus and reevaluate the stability of the first ray and motion between the medial and middle cuneiform on stress views under fluoroscopy. If there is any intercuneiform instability, then proceeding to a true Lapidus procedure is necessary.
- Nonunion, malunion, and shortening have been worrisome complications of the Lapidus procedures for decades. However, with the progress in understanding of the anatomy, function, and biomechanical characteristics of the first tarsometatarsal joint, substantial development in both surgical approaches and new fixation techniques has been made. Some fixation methods, such as a plantar plate, nitinol staples, and intramedullary fixation, have been proven to be stronger biomechanically in cadaveric studies.

First tarsometatarsal (TMT) joint arthrodesis was introduced to treat hallux valgus deformity at the beginning of the last century[1–3] and then was popularized by Lapidus[4] in the 1950s with a focus on indications for correction of hallux valgus associated with first ray hypermobility. When Lapidus introduced the procedure, the focus was only on

Steps2Walk, 1209 Harbor Island Walk, Baltimore, MD 21230, USA
* Corresponding author.
E-mail address: drshuyuanli@gmail.com

Foot Ankle Clin N Am 25 (2020) 109–126
https://doi.org/10.1016/j.fcl.2019.11.001
1083-7515/20/© 2019 Elsevier Inc. All rights reserved.

foot.theclinics.com

a single plane of instability in the sagittal plane, associated with presumed first TMT joint hypermobility, which had already been recognized as a source of dysfunction of both the forefoot and the midfoot, including hallux valgus, lesser metatarsalgia, stress fracture of the lesser metatarsals, and midfoot arthritis.[5–7] Since that time, the Lapidus procedure has been used in treating failed or recurrent hallux valgus surgeries (**Fig. 1**),[8] hallux varus deformity, and metatarsal adductus (**Fig. 2**)[9] as well as hindfoot deformity (**Fig. 3**), all with good results.

During the past several decades, many modifications have been introduced into the technical aspects of both the procedure and the methods of fixation in order to improve the outcome and reduce complications. In this article, the authors discuss why the Lapidus procedure is necessary, differentiate the importance of the classic Lapidus and modified Lapidus procedures, and then elaborate on the development of different methods of fixation that have accompanied the evolution of this procedure.

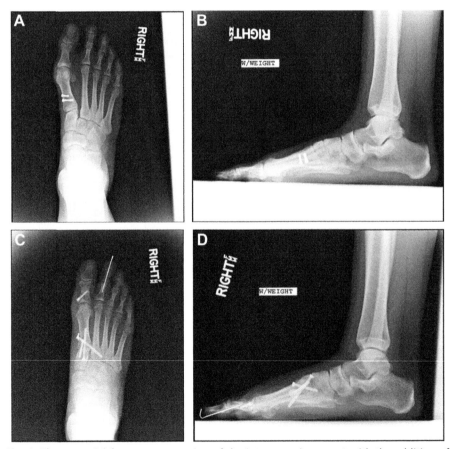

Fig. 1. The potential for overcompression of the interspace is present with the addition of the intermetatarsal screw. Note in this case (*A, B*) (a revision hallux valgus surgery) that the distal head of the metatarsal appears to be facing slightly laterally. This can easily occur with compression of the oblique Lapidus screw. It is possible that the appearance here could have been improved by further supinating the metatarsal (*C, D*).

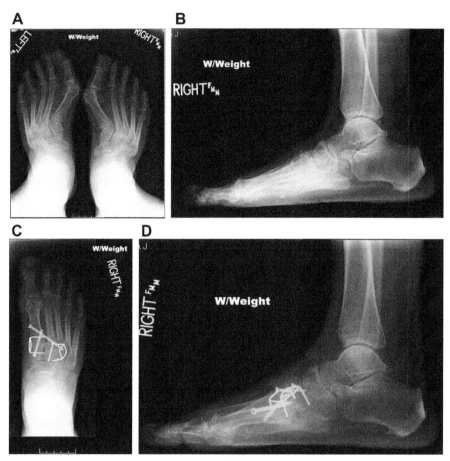

Fig. 2. Metatarsus adductus is an unusually difficult deformity to manage with a standard metatarsal osteotomy, and even so, when the lesser metatarsals are corrected into abduction (*A, B*), there remains a large intermetatarsal angle, which can be treated with a variety of methods of fixation, here with a combination of screws and nitinol staples (*C, D*).

WHY IS IT NECESSARY TO FUSE THE FIRST TARSOMETATARSAL JOINT?

First TMT joint instability has been found to be a main cause of both primary and recurrent hallux valgus. According to a systematic review and metaanalysis evaluating the difference in the first ray range of motion between patients with or without hallux valgus deformity, there was a significant 3.62-mm increase of first ray sagittal motion in patients with hallux valgus deformity compared with those without hallux valgus deformity.[10] In a retrospective review study of 32 feet treated with the Lapidus procedure for recurrent hallux valgus, preoperative evaluation revealed that 96% of patients had clinical hypermobility of the first TMT joint and 52% had radiographic findings of instability.[8] One must not however focus on hypermobility of the first metatarsal as the reason to perform this procedure. Certainly, there are cases in which hypermobility is obvious, and not only is the first metatarsal excessively mobile in dorsiflexion, but there is clinical overload of the lesser metatarsals characterized by metatarsalgia,

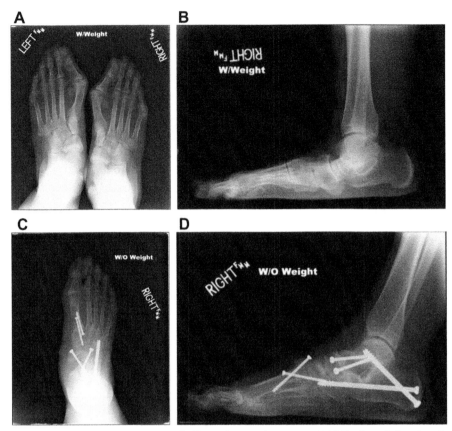

Fig. 3. Associated with a recurrent hallux valgus and a severe rigid flatfoot deformity, the modified Lapidus in addition to a triple arthrodesis is a good procedure (*A, B*). Given the length of time of immobilization following the triple arthrodesis, this screw configuration remains acceptable (*C, D*).

stress fractures of the lesser metatarsals, or arthritis of the second and third TMT joints (**Fig. 4**).

Correcting First Tarsometatarsal Hypermobility in Both Sagittal and Transversal Planes

Hypermobility of the first metatarsal in the sagittal plane has been recognized to be only one of the pathologic indications for the procedure because increased mobility in the transverse plane is just as important. According to Faber and colleagues[11,12] in a biomechanical study, first TMT joint hypermobility occurred in both the sagittal and the transversal planes. Therefore, when considering a Lapidus procedure for surgically correcting a hallux valgus, the mobility of the first metatarsal in the transverse plane should also be assessed. Transverse plane instability can be diagnosed by strapping the forefoot with tape and then taking weight-bearing anteroposterior radiographs. If the alignment of the first metatarsal is reduced through taping, then there is instability in the transverse plane, and a Lapidus procedure is likely to be indicated (**Fig. 5**).[12,13]

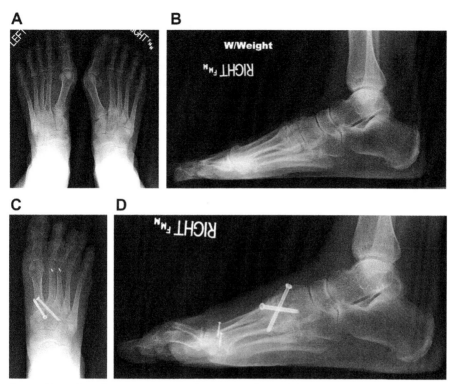

Fig. 4. This patient does not appear to have a significant deformity, but the association of a stress fracture at the base of the second metatarsal (*A, B*) indicates substantial overload requiring a Lapidus procedure (*C, D*). The fixation is not optimal, and although this sufficed to stabilize the base of the second metatarsal and treat the stress fracture with crossed screw and cancellous grafting, the fixation of the first metatarsal is not correct.

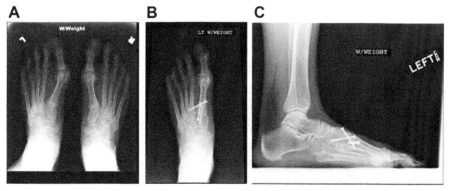

Fig. 5. A moderate deformity with bilateral TMT instability (*A*). Transverse plane instability was confirmed by strapping the forefoot with tape (not shown). The method of fixation of the Lapidus procedure is quite adequate. The question arises as to the need for debridement of bone grafting in between the first and second metatarsal, a procedure which the authors advocate (*B, C*).

Correcting Hallux Valgus Three-Dimensionally

For decades, little attention has been paid to the need to rotate or supinate the first metatarsal in the frontal plane. Although the correction of the intermetatarsal angle has been adequate following either Lapidus procedure, unless the sesamoids are perfectly reduced under the metatarsal head, and in particular, if the metatarsal stays slightly pronated, recurrent hallux valgus will likely occur. In recent years, more and more attention has been paid to the 3-dimensional changes in hallux valgus deformity.[14] Singh and colleagues[15] compared the first ray hypermobility in both dorsal and dorsomedial direction between feet with and without hallux valgus. They reported that in the group without hallux valgus, there were a mean of 7.2-mm (4.2–11.3) displacement in the dorsal direction (sagittal plane) and a mean of 8.3-mm (4.0–12.6) displacement in the 45° dorsomedial direction, whereas in the hallux valgus group, there was 9.8-mm (5.2–14.1) displacement in the dorsal direction and a mean of 11.0-mm (5.9–16.2) displacement in the 45° dorsomedial direction. They proposed that the traditional measurement of the first ray hypermobility only in the sagittal plane, and the hallux valgus angle and intermetatarsal angle only in transversal plane were not reasonable. Because there could be far more movement in multiple planes, measurement of the first ray hypermobility in a 45° dorsomedial direction was more appropriate. The first metatarsal pronation plays a very important role in the cause of hallux valgus deformity. It can cause radiological artifact changes, such as a pronated first metatarsal head with an everted lateral condyle is often confused with a large distal metatarsal articular angle, and in some cases, the lateral shifting of both sesamoids together with the first metatarsal head pronation can be mistakenly interpreted as sesamoid subluxation.[16,17] According to the authors' experience, the unaddressed first metatarsal pronation will quite likely lead to failure of a procedure sooner or later even if the intermetatarsal angle is well reduced (**Fig. 6**).

Among the current hallux valgus deformity correction surgeries, the Lapidus procedures have a strong capability to derotate the pronated first metatarsal and reduce the subluxated sesamoids. This is because most of the rotation (pronation) occurs at the TMT joint. Dayton and colleagues[18] observed in a case series study that there was a consistent valgus, or everted position of the first metatarsal as a component of the hallux valgus deformity, which was corrected by varus rotation or inversion of the first metatarsal after a modified Lapidus procedure, with a 10.1° reduction of the

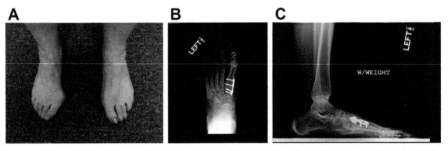

A   B   C

Fig. 6. Although the intermetatarsal angle in this case is reduced to almost 0°, why is the hallux in valgus? (*A*). Note the presence of the fibular sesamoid indicating that the first metatarsal was never supinated during the procedure (*B, C*). Adding an Akin osteotomy "cheats" the surgeon into thinking that the rotation of the hallux is corrected, but this never is the case because the rotation is more proximal than the hallux.

intermetatarsal angle, a 17.8° reduction of the hallux abductus angle, an 18.7° change in the proximal articular set angle, and a change of 3.8 in the tibial sesamoid position. In another study, Dayton and colleagues[19] observed that the amount of first metatarsal frontal plane rotation (supination) needed to anatomically align the first TMT joint on an anterior posterior radiograph without soft tissue balancing was a mean of 22.1° ± 5.2° supination rotation. This was performed during the Lapidus procedure by achieving a mean amount of 6.9° ± 3.0° intermetatarsal angle reduction and a mean amount of 3.3° ± 1.2° of the tibial sesamoid position. Moreover, univariate linear regression analysis showed that greater preoperative tibial sesamoid position scores were associated with greater intraoperative supination rotation required for joint alignment. These studies (without doing distal soft tissue release) further strengthened the notion that the frontal plane rotation plays an important role in the hallux valgus deformity.[19]

Biomechanical Benefits of the Lapidus Procedures

The Lapidus procedure is performed closest to the apex of the deformity. Although this does not correspond to the center of rotation angle, which is generally located more proximally than the first TMT joint in the proximal aspect of the medial cuneiform or even the navicular, theoretically the Lapidus procedure has a stronger power than other procedures to correct hallux valgus deformity. A metaanalysis of 29 studies with a total of 1470 operated feet showed the first TMT arthrodesis had higher corrective power compared with metaanalysis data on proximal, diaphyseal, and distal metatarsal osteotomies.[20]

The Lapidus arthrodesis may also help strengthen the medial longitudinal arch. A cadaveric study observed significant frontal plane eversion of the medial and dorsiflexion of the talus occurred after Lapidus arthrodesis was performed, which suggested that arthrodesis at the first TMT joint increased the efficiency of the peroneal longus and its stabilizing action on the medial column.[21] Similar results were also reported clinically that after performing a modified Lapidus procedure, the talo-first metatarsal angle and medial cuneiform height both had statistically significant increases, 2.97° and 3.44 mm, respectively.[22] Another study using both radiographic and pedobarographic evaluation observed that the Lapidus procedure reduced hallux plantar pressure significantly; however, the Lapidus group also exhibited a significant increase in the mean fifth metatarsal head plantar pressure and pressure under the fifth metatarsal as a percentage of the total forefoot, which means that the Lapidus arthrodesis may have greater influence on the load-sharing distribution of forefoot pressure.[23] It was also proven on a 3-dimensional finite element foot model that the first TMT joint arthrodesis could increase the stress on the first metatarsal and reduce the stress on the second metatarsal in both midstance and push-off phases and reduce medial excursion of the first metatarsal head, that is, restore the load-bearing function of the first ray.[24]

WHEN DO YOU NEED A TRADITIONAL LAPIDUS PROCEDURE?

The most important distinction between the original Lapidus and the modified Lapidus is the arthrodesis between the first and second rays which is performed in the original Lapidus procedure while not in the modified Lapidus procedure. Regardless of the method of fixation for each, these are 2 completely different procedures and have different implications for outcome and function. A traditional Lapidus has been criticized for causing too much stiffness, which can cause overload on the first ray in particular under the sesamoids (**Fig. 7**). A modified Lapidus procedure, on the other hand, allows for slight sagittal plane motion in the medial column, and this can permit

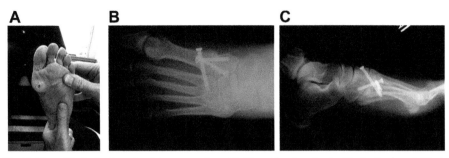

Fig. 7. The effect of a true Lapidus procedure (*A*, *B*) on the forefoot with limited mobility in the sagittal plane, in particular, in dorsiflexion, in this case producing increased pressure under the sesamoid, causing a plantar callosity and pain. Note the plantarflexed first metatarsal on the lateral view of the radiograph (*B*) and the plantar callosity underneath the sesamoids (*C*).

offloading of the sesamoids in the event of a rigid metatarsal. This is particularly relevant if a true Lapidus procedure has been performed and a plantar or dorsal malunion occurs leading to overload of either the sesamoids or the second metatarsal. Therefore, during the procedure, the authors always prefer to perform a modified Lapidus first. However, too much mobility between the first and second metatarsals and between the medial and middle cuneiform can lead to recurrent deformity as a result of increasing varus of the metatarsal as the metatarsal drifts off medially away from the second metatarsal. This evolution of thinking is presented in a paragraph by John Anderson, MD and his colleagues at Orthopedic Associates in Grand Rapids, Michigan.

"Initially, two screws placed across the first TMT were used. After realizing that several metatarsus primus varus cases recurred, even after the first TMT joint solidly fused, it was obvious that the 1 to 2 inter cuneiform joint was a source of recurrent deformity and we started using a transverse screw to hold this interval stable, but did not do anything to try to fuse this interval, rather simply used a screw to try to hold it stable. The screw eventually was removed or broke because of micro motion, and in most was not a problem but in some we saw recurrent metatarsus varus with recurrent hallux valgus. Recurrent metatarsus varus should not occur if the first TMT heals, unless there is another source of motion. No current bunion technique involving osteotomies addresses the 1 to 2 interval. Our current technique is to burr and denude the 1 to 2 interspace between the proximal first and second metatarsals, and the distal aspect of the 1 to 2 intercuneiform joint and bone graft with local bone graft or allograft, and hold with transverse screws between the first and second metatarsals and the first and second cuneiforms, and try to obtain a spot weld between the first and second rays. This theoretically makes it mathematically impossible for recurrent metatarsus primus varus. In reality, it has reduced our recurrence to near zero. Technique is critical and fusion principles apply (remove soft tissues, prepare bone, drill for bleeding, rigid fixation). The additional screws have enhanced stability, so we now allow heel WBAT at 2 weeks in a boot and start early ROM and use only boots, not casts, and the early WB has not reduced our first TMT fusion rate, rather it has increased it, to close to 99%. I have now used more than two transverse screws when worried about bone stability or bone quality, as intercuneiform instability has become a primary source of recurrent deformity, and more metal has always been my solution for slow healing" (John Anderson, MD, personal communication, 2017).

In a cadaveric study, the sagittal plane motion of the first ray was 7.45 ± 1.82 mm before fusing the first TMT joint, but with isolated first TMT joint fusion with a crossed screw technique, the sagittal motion decreased to 4.41 ± 1.51 mm and decreased significantly further to 3.12 ± 1.06 mm, with the addition of middle cuneiform fixation. This suggested that first ray to second ray fixation can be beneficial and necessary if excessive sagittal motion is present after isolated first TMT joint arthrodesis.[25]

The authors' experience is that after completing the modified Lapidus, the stability of the first ray and motion between the medial and middle cuneiform are always reevaluated on stress view under fluoroscopy. If there is any intercuneiform instability, then it is necessary to proceed to a true Lapidus procedure (**Fig. 8**).

COMPLICATIONS OF LAPIDUS PROCEDURES
Nonunion, Malunion

For decades, the higher rate of nonunion has been a concern associated with the Lapidus procedure. The reported nonunion rate was as high as 6% to 12%.[26–28] Although radiographic nonunion is the most frequent complication, probably only 25% to 50% of the patients with this condition have associated clinical findings.[29] Malunion and dorsal elevation of the first metatarsal are other common complications, which could lead to dysfunction of the first ray and overloading of the lesser metatarsals. The high rate of nonunion and malunion in the 1990s may have some relationship to the unstable methods of screw fixation used at that time.[7]

Joint preparation and correct positioning are very important steps, which are relevant to the outcome of the procedure. To some extent, nonunion may have had to do with the method of joint preparation in addition to the type of fixation used. Joint preparation by debridement with preservation of the subchondral bone plate has the advantage of preserving the length of the metatarsal. Originally, the joint was debrided down to the subchondral bone and then perforated with a 2-mm drill. In the early 2000s, the authors' method of preparation of the joint changed with much more aggressive chiseling and perforation to create a bone slurry in the joint, which seemed to increase the rate of arthrodesis. The only potential problem with this method of joint preparation is that it leads to multiple "spot welding" of the joint,

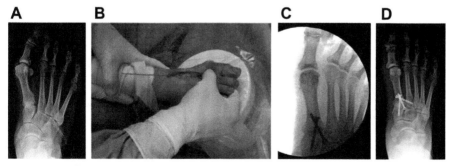

Fig. 8. A modified Lapidus procedure was used to correct this moderate hallux valgus deformity with first TMT joint instability (A). During the surgery, after the first TMT joint was fixed with 2 screws, a stress test was done under fluoroscopy by squeezing the intermetatarsal space between the first and second ray (B). Intercuneiform instability was noted with gapping between the first and second metatarsals (C). The surgery was therefore converted into a true Lapidus procedure by adding a screw in between the first and second metatarsal while the metatarsals were held reduced (D).

which is not the case with a straight saw cut. Although free-hand straight saw cuts had the advantage of providing a smoother bone apposition, this was also associated with a risk of removing too much bone from the curved-shaped joint, shortening the metatarsal, and ultimately causing overload of the lateral metatarsals. It needs to be realized that through lateral translation, plantar flexion, and supination of the first metatarsal head, the first metatarsus varus and pronation deformity will be addressed nicely without taking out any extra bone. A retrospective study with radiograph and chart review on 110 feet that underwent a first TMT joint arthrodesis for primary Hallux valgus (HV) angle correction using a curettage technique without wedge resection showed that that kind of procedure had a significant ability to correct the first intermetatarsal angle, HV angle, and tibial sesamoid position.[30] A major change with joint preparation has come with the introduction of precise saw cuts using specific cutting guides to prepare the joint introduced by Paragon28 (Englewood, CO, USA) and Treace Medical.

Results from a recent systematic review analyzing 8 studies and 443 arthrodeses demonstrated a nonunion rate of 3.61%.[31] This may be due to improvement in fixation method, joint preparation techniques, and a better understanding of both anatomic structure and biomechanical function of the first TMT joint in the recent years.

Shortening

Shortening was a potentially serious complication after the Lapidus procedure caused by a flat saw cut or a closing wedge cut, whereby too much bone had been removed (**Fig. 9**). The literature reports a shortening around 5 mm after fusing the first TMT joint.[28,32] First metatarsal bone shortening is associated with lesser metatarsal overloading and metatarsalgia. In order to prevent this, intentional plantar flexion of the first metatarsal or using bone graft during the arthrodesis was suggested. However, surgeons should realize that there is a limitation to the plantar flexion of the first metatarsal, because too much plantar flexion could lead to overloading and sesamoid pain. Furthermore, as the plantarflexion of the first metatarsal increases, the hallux becomes dysfunctional by extending at the metatarsophalangeal joint, and with the ensuing extensor hallucis longus contracture, pushes the metatarsal into even more plantarflexion. Bone grafting of the arthrodesis can achieve about 50% reduction of the original shortening.[28,32] Therefore, the most ideal way to prevent shortening is to do a rotational first TMT joint fusion by only removing the joint surface and keeping the curved shape of the joint.

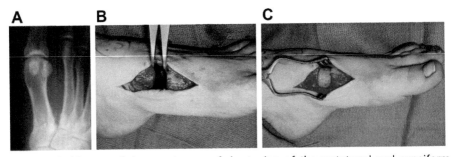

Fig. 9. Probably one of the worst cases of shortening of the metatarsal and cuneiform following a Lapidus procedure, where a saw was used to remove too much bone off both the metatarsal and the cuneiform (A). This led to overload of the second metatarsal and was resolved by insertion of a large tricortical structural bone graft to restore length (B, C).

Recurrence of Hallux Valgus Deformity

Recurrence is another complication that can occur in cases with poor fixation or insufficient addressed multiple plantar hypermobility whereby a true Lapidus instead of a modified Lapidus procedure should have been done.[33] As noted above, probably the most common cause and the one least recognized is inadequate derotation (supination) of the metatarsal.

WHAT ARE IDEAL METHODS OF FIXATION

Surgeons face a variety of challenges and complications in correction with a Lapidus procedure. The first is prominence of hardware, creating patient discomfort, occurring whether dorsally plated or with screws, particularly under the more vulnerable dorsal skin. Generation and maintenance of compression at fusion site to allow for primary healing are not possible with many of the screw or screw and plate configurations available. Gapping of one of the surfaces of the joint, whether plantar, medial, or lateral, will inevitably lead to some sort of failure of correction of deformity.

When talking about fixation, there are 2 things that need to be considered: the first is if a traditional Lapidus is necessary, and then, second, what kind of fixation method for the first TMT joint could provide a high union rate and early postoperative mobility. As has been discussed earlier, if following the first TMT fusion, there is still obvious instability between the first and second rays under stress fluoroscopy, a true Lapidus procedure is then indicated. Also noted earlier is the performance of a true Lapidus procedure as a routine by some surgeons with a high success rate (no recurrence and a high rate of arthrodesis). There remains the concern for the optimal fixation of the first to the second ray.

Crossed Screws

The use of screws across the joint has been the traditional, and the most inexpensive and frequently used technique for fixation, but not the most reliable. Following compression with 1 partially threaded screw, there is compression that ranges from 30 to 40 N. If 2 compression screws are used across the joint, will this increase the amount of compression? If 1 screw compresses the joint, the second compression screw will only lead to slight loosening of the first screw and loss of compression. This could theoretically be minimized by tightening the first screw, but the authors' experience has been that this is less than ideal. The second option, and one that the authors support, is to use 1 compression screw, and then, if they are using screws only for fixation, the second screw is fully threaded to maximize purchase, but not to add any further compression. In order to gain maximum purchase and avoid any screw prominence, the authors use a burr to create the countersink for the screw head. The first screw is introduced from proximal to distal, and the burr hole is made in the middle of the cuneiform slightly laterally. This allows for plenty of room to introduce the second screw from distal to proximal where the burr hole is made 1 cm distal to the joint but slightly medial on the metatarsal and where the authors advocate the use of a fully threaded screw. The compression that is obtained with this screw technique is not sufficient, and ideally 80 to 100 N is required for optimal compression at the first TMT joint. Screw fixation that is in more than 1 plane does not increase the stability of the arthrodesis construct, although in **Fig. 4**, this was acceptable because of the stress fracture of the base of the second metatarsal treated with cancellous bone grafting and the oblique screw as noted.

This does not mean however that crossed screws can be used indiscriminately, expecting arthrodesis to take place. In **Fig. 10**, the screw technique used is

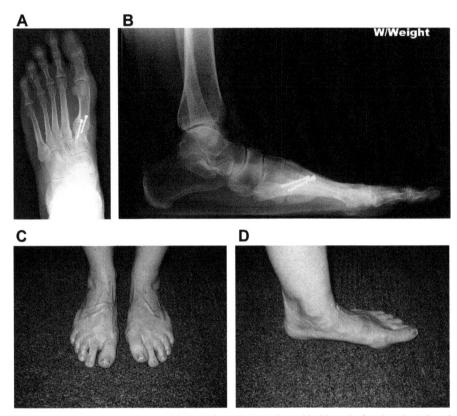

Fig. 10. The screw technique used here is hopeless, with no likelihood of arthrodesis (*A–D*). Furthermore, the metatarsal has been left pronated, which then leads to recurrence of the hallux valgus, and because insufficient bone has been removed from the plantar surface of the joint, there is a dorsal malunion present. These findings are evident in the radiographs as well and the clinical images with a cock-up hallux, recurrent hallux valgus, and elevation of the first metatarsal.

hopeless, with no likelihood of arthrodesis. Furthermore, the metatarsal has been left pronated, which then leads to recurrence of the hallux valgus, and because insufficient bone has been removed from the plantar surface of the joint, there is a dorsal malunion present.

Plate Fixation

Plate fixation is another alternative fixation method. Although a plate can be placed dorsally, dorsomedially, medially, or on the plantar surface, it is now widely thought that a single compression screw dorsally supplemented by a medial plate with added potential for compression increases the biomechanical advantage of fixation, stability, and resistance to load bearing in the sagittal and transverse plane. Not only does a dorsal plating system fail to confer any mechanical advantage but also it has been demonstrated in a cadaveric study that the dorsal plating technique had a higher risk of damaging surrounding blood vessels and nerves. In contrast, medial plating is safe without injury to the insertion of the tibialis anterior muscle or the saphenous and superficial fibular nerves.[34]

Plating Plus a Lag Screw

In addition to placing a plate, using a compression screw across the first TMT joint may provide more stability and a high union rate and allow for an early postoperative mobilization. In cadavers, the mean time to 50% peak compression for "plate-with-lag-screw" construct was 3 times that of the "plate-only" construct.[35] A cohort study in 59 feet among 58 patients showed this kind of fixation technique could achieve a mean of 7 weeks postoperative protected full weight-bearing, 98.31% bony union, and a 94.12% patient satisfactory rate.[36]

Similar biomechanical findings were reported in different orientations of placing the compression screw. In a cadaver study, it was found that using a same low-profile locking plate technique but by changing the additional screw from an intraplate compression screw into a plantar interfragmentary screw placed on the tension side of the arthrodesis significantly increased the stability of the Lapidus arthrodesis fixation construct.[37] The same team further observed biomechanical stability difference in using the same plantar-distal to dorsal-proximal compression screw technique but changing the plate fixation from a medially applied low-profile into a plantarly applied anatomic locking plate. There was no significant difference found between the 2 groups with respect to ultimate load to failure, stiffness of the construct, or moment at time of failure.[38]

The system of Paragon28 has been a clinically very reliable method of fixation, taking advantage of the dorsal compression screw, supplemented by a unique plantar tab that maximizes fixation of the construct. The Lapidus Arthrodesis System was developed around the concept of neutralization plating. A plate designed for the medial wall provides added stiffness because the plate is positioned on its side. Traditionally, medial wall plates can complicate the fixation because the distal screws apply a medializing (adduction) force on the first metatarsal as they are tightened to the plate. To combat this, the plate was designed to match the corrected metatarsal position as well as the local curvature, thus following the principles of a "bent plate technique" to limit the transverse plane force applied to the metatarsal (**Fig. 11**). In addition, a medial wall plate is better positioned to prevent plantar gapping while avoiding the insertion of the tibialis anterior plantarly. The anatomic plate construct is designed to help reduce soft tissue irritation in an area where ample soft tissue coverage can be a concern with a poorly designed plate construct. Two very useful additional features include a plantar locking arm to better resist the tension side of the joint, and a precision guide for crossing dorsal compression screw insertion to avoid collision with the locking plate screws. The plate screw configuration is a perfect method of fixation as part of the reconstruction of a flatfoot deformity (**Fig. 12**).

Staple Fixation

Nitinol compression staples provide yet another choice for fixation. The presumed advantage of nitinol staples is the continued compression that is maintained following insertion of the staple compared with screw fixation where there is immediate loss of compression. A biomechanical study using saw bone models observed mechanical changes in crossed screws, claw plate, single staple, or double staple constructs, when being contoured to 1, 2, and 3 mm of plantar displacement.[39] Results showed that both single- and double-staple constructs induced a significantly greater contact force and area across the arthrodesis than the crossed screw-and-claw plate constructs at all measurements. The staple constructs completely recovered their plantar gapping following each test. The claw plate generated the least contact force and area at the joint interface and had significantly greater plantar

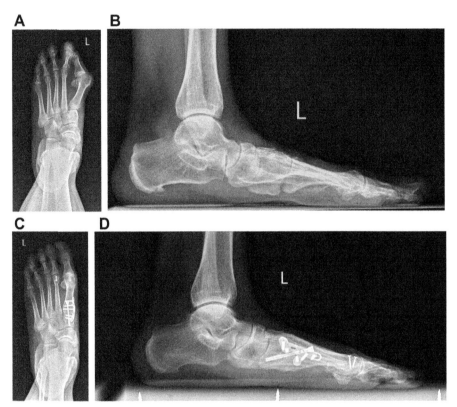

Fig. 11. The metatarsal is quite unstable in both the sagittal and the transverse plane (*A, B*). Note the gapping of the plantar aspect of the first TMT joint (*B*). The use of a medial plate for fixation of the Lapidus fusion has the advantage of the precision guide, which allows the insertion of the compression screw dorsally, but no overlapping screws medially. The medial plate application is biomechanically very stable and permits early bearing of weight. Note the screw and plate construct and the early arthrodesis (*C, D*). Note however persistent sub-luxation of the sesamoids, an ominous sign with respect to incomplete rotation of the first metatarsal and a higher incidence of recurrence (*C*). (*Courtesy of* Thomas San Giovanni, MD, Coral Gables, FL.)

gapping than all other constructs and probably should be avoided with the mechanically more stable methods of fixation available today. The crossed screw constructs were significantly stiffer and had significantly less plantar gapping than the other constructs, but this gapping was not recoverable. Crossed screw fixation provides a rigid arthrodesis with limited compression and contact footprint across the joint. Shape memory alloy staples afford dynamic fixation with sustained compression across the arthrodesis.

Intramedullary Fixation

The Lapidus Intramedullary Nail (Paragon28) features a zero-prominence implant, which can eliminate the pain associated with hardware prominence in traditional plating systems. From a biomechanical perspective, the nail can withstand greater forces across the fusion site and limits migration during healing to facilitate potential earlier weight-bearing. Being intramedullary, the nail is capable of accepting greater

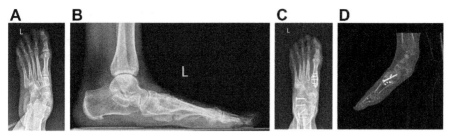

Fig. 12. Although the hallux valgus and intermetatarsal angle are not severe, note the insta-bility of the first TMT joint with gapping on the plantar surface (*A*, *B*), in a case with classic features requiring a Lapidus procedure. Note plantar gapping of the first TMT joint, severe deformity associated with uncovering of the talonavicular joint, and a severe flatfoot defor-mity. The overall alignment following correction is perfect, with the sesamoids well located under the metatarsal head, indicating good derotation of the first metatarsal with reduc-tion of the intermetatarsal angle and the hallux valgus (*C*). The flatfoot has been well cor-rected following lateral column lengthening plus the Lapidus procedure (*C*, *D*). (Case courtesy of Thomas San Giovanni, MD, Coral Gables, FL.)

forces across the fusion site and limits migration during healing while providing even compression across the first TMT joint.

This limitation of forces across the fusion site is important to understand with respect to crossed screws and alternate plating systems. For example, a medially applied plate is best able to resist a dorsoplantar force, whereas an intramedullary nail can resist forces in 3 planes, including rotation, dorsal as well as mediolateral bending.

The Paragon28 Nail has crossed screw fixation distally, and the proportionate amount of force that the nail exerts in all directions resists recurrent hallux valgus. One of the better features is a calibrated compression driver so surgeons can deter-mine when the nail has achieved ideal compression. The nail comes in lengths of 38 to 60 mm and has threaded pegs for bicortical fixation and threading through the nail proximally and then distally following compression (**Fig. 13**).

HOW TO PLACE THE FIRST AND SECOND RAY FIXATION

The multiple plane instability between the first and second rays is still poorly under-stood. It could occur in between the first and second metatarsals, the first and second cuneiforms, or both. As a result, there has been no definite instruction for how to place

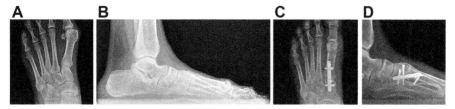

Fig. 13. Note the presence of gross instability of the first metatarsal with marked elevatus and instability of the first TMT joint (*A*, *B*). This has been extremely well corrected using an intramedullary nail. Note the perfect reduction in the anteroposterior view as well as the correction of the elevated metatarsal (*C*, *D*). (Case courtesy of Leonard Vekkos, DPM, Woodridge, IL.)

the first and second ray fixation. It was found in a cadaveric study that stability of the first ray in the transverse and coronal planes was not improved with TMT joint fixation alone or with an additional first to second cuneiform screw. The first to second metatarsal screw consistently reduced first metatarsal instability in both planes. The first metatarsal to middle cuneiform screw had intermediate results.[40]

SUMMARY

In general, the evolution of Lapidus fixation has been strongly associated with the understanding of the anatomy and function of the first TMT joint, the mechanism of hypermobility of the first TMT joint, and cause of the hallux valgus deformity in 3 dimensions. Progress in those above aspects has substantially promoted the development of new fixation techniques. A stable fixation will reduce the rate of nonunion and allow for early postoperative weight-bearing. The decision of whether to perform an original Lapidus or a modified Lapidus can be made intraoperatively after the first TMT joint has been fused and the stability between the first and second rays has been reevaluated under stress test. Alternatively, because some authors have incorporated (John Anderson, MD, personal communication) this as part of their routine method of fixation, further clinical studies are needed to examine whether current biomechanical study findings could bring relevant clinical outcomes.

DISCLOSURE

Dr S. Li has nothing to disclose. Dr M.S. Myerson is a Consultant for Paragon 28.

REFERENCES

1. Truslow W. Metatarsus primus varus or hallux valgus? J Bone Joint Surg Am 1925; 7:98.
2. Kleinberg S. Operative cure of hallux valgus and bunions. Am J Surg 1932;15: 75–81.
3. Espinosa N, Wirth SH. Unstable first ray and failed bunion surgery. Foot Ankle Clin 2011;16(1):21–34.
4. Lapidus PW. A quarter of a century of experience with the operative correction of the metatarsus varus primus in hallux valgus. Bull Hosp Joint Dis 1956;17(2): 404–21.
5. Maguire W. The Lapidus procedure for hallux valgus. J Bone Joint Surg Br 1973; 55:221.
6. Klaue K, Hansen ST, Masquelet AC. Clinical, quantitative assessment of first tarsometatarsal mobility in the sagittal plane and its relation to hallux valgus deformity. Foot Ankle Int 1994;15(1):9–13.
7. Johnson KA, Kile TA. Hallux valgus due to cuneiform-metatarsal instability. J South Orthop Assoc 1994;3(4):273–82.
8. Ellington JK, Myerson MS, Coetzee JC, et al. The use of the Lapidus procedure for recurrent hallux valgus. Foot Ankle Int 2011;32(7):674–80.
9. Aiyer A, Shub J, Shariff R, et al. Radiographic recurrence of deformity after hallux valgus surgery in patients with metatarsus adductus. Foot Ankle Int 2016;37(2): 165–71.
10. Shibuya N, Roukis TS, Jupiter DC. Mobility of the first ray in patients with or without hallux valgus deformity: systematic review and meta-analysis. J Foot Ankle Surg 2017;56(5):1070–5.

11. Faber FW, Kleinrensink GJ, Verhoog MW, et al. Mobility of the first tarsometatarsal joint in relation to hallux valgus deformity: anatomical and biomechanical aspects. Foot Ankle Int 1999;20(10):651–6.

12. Myerson MS, Kadakia AR. The Lapidus procedure. Reconstructive foot and ankle surgery: management of complications. 3rd edition. Philadelphia: Elsevier; 2018. p. 13–26.

13. Romash MM, Fugate D, Yanklowit B. Passive motion of the first metatarsal cuneiform joint: preoperative assessment. Foot Ankle 1990;10(6):293–8.

14. Dayton P, Kauwe M, Feilmeier M. Is our current paradigm for evaluation and management of the bunion deformity flawed? A discussion of procedure philosophy relative to anatomy. J Foot Ankle Surg 2015;54(1):102–11.

15. Singh D, Biz C, Corradin M, et al. Comparison of dorsal and dorsomedial displacement in evaluation of first ray hypermobility in feet with and without hallux valgus. Foot Ankle Surg 2016;22(2):120–4.

16. Dayton P, Feilmeier M. Comparison of tibial sesamoid position on anteroposterior and axial radiographs before and after triplane tarsal metatarsal joint arthrodesis. J Foot Ankle Surg 2017;56(5):1041–6.

17. Santrock RD, Smith B. Hallux valgus deformity and treatment: a three-dimensional approach: modified technique for Lapidus procedure. Foot Ankle Clin 2018;23(2):281–95.

18. Dayton P, Feilmeier M, Kauwe M, et al. Relationship of frontal plane rotation of first metatarsal to proximal articular set angle and hallux alignment in patients undergoing tarsometatarsal arthrodesis for hallux abducto valgus: a case series and critical review of the literature. J Foot Ankle Surg 2013;52(3):348–54.

19. Dayton P, Kauwe M, DiDomenico L, et al. Quantitative analysis of the degree of frontal rotation required to anatomically align the first metatarsal phalangeal joint during modified tarsal-metatarsal arthrodesis without capsular balancing. J Foot Ankle Surg 2016;55(2):220–5.

20. Willegger M, Holinka J, Ristl R, et al. Correction power and complications of first tarsometatarsal joint arthrodesis for hallux valgus deformity. Int Orthop 2015; 39(3):467–76.

21. Bierman RA, Christensen JC, Johnson CH. Biomechanics of the first ray. Part III. Consequences of Lapidus arthrodesis on peroneus longus function: a three-dimensional kinematic analysis in a cadaver model. J Foot Ankle Surg 2001; 40(3):125–31.

22. Avino A, Patel S, Hamilton GA, et al. The effect of the Lapidus arthrodesis on the medial longitudinal arch: a radiographic review. J Foot Ankle Surg 2008;47(6): 510–4.

23. King CM, Hamilton GA, Ford LA. Effects of the lapidus arthrodesis and chevron bunionectomy on plantar forefoot pressures. J Foot Ankle Surg 2014;53(4):415–9.

24. Wai-Chi Wong D, Wang Y, Zhang M, et al. Functional restoration and risk of nonunion of the first metatarsocuneiform arthrodesis for hallux valgus: a finite element approach. J Biomech 2015;48(12):3142–8.

25. Galli MM, McAlister JE, Berlet GC, et al. Enhanced Lapidus arthrodesis: crossed screw technique with middle cuneiform fixation further reduces sagittal mobility. J Foot Ankle Surg 2015;54(3):437–40.

26. Myerson MS. Metatarsocuneiform arthrodesis for treatment of hallux valgus and metatarsus primus varus. Orthopedics 1990;13(9):1025–31.

27. Myerson M, Allon S, McGarvey W. Metatarsocuneiform arthrodesis for management of hallux valgus and metatarsus primus varus. Foot Ankle 1992;13:107–15.

28. Catanzariti AR, Mendicino RW, Lee MS, et al. The modified Lapidus arthrodesis: a retrospective analysis. J Foot Ankle Surg 1999;38(5):322–32.
29. Myerson MS, Badekas A. Hypermobility of the first ray. Foot Ankle Clin 2000;5(3):469–84.
30. McAlister JE, Peterson KS, Hyer CF. Corrective realignment arthrodesis of the first tarsometatarsal joint without wedge resection. Foot Ankle Spec 2015;8(4):284–8.
31. Crowell A, Van JC, Meyr AJ. Early weightbearing after arthrodesis of the first metatarsal-medial cuneiform joint: a systematic review of the incidence of nonunion. J Foot Ankle Surg 2018;57(6):1204–6.
32. Fleming L, Savage TJ, Paden MH, et al. Results of modified lapidus arthrodesis procedure using medial eminence as an interpositional autograft. J Foot Ankle Surg 2011;50(3):272–5.
33. Bednarz PA, Manoli A 2nd. Modified lapidus procedure for the treatment of hypermobile hallux valgus. Foot Ankle Int 2000;21(10):816–21.
34. Simons P, Fröber R, Loracher C, et al. First tarsometatarsal arthrodesis: an anatomic evaluation of dorsomedial versus plantar plating. J Foot Ankle Surg 2015;54(5):787–92.
35. Garas PK, DiSegna ST, Patel AR. Plate alone versus plate and lag screw for lapidus arthrodesis: a biomechanical comparison of compression. Foot Ankle Spec 2018;11(6):534–8.
36. Klos K, Wilde CH, Lange A, et al. Modified lapidus arthrodesis with plantar plate and compression screw for treatment of hallux valgus with hypermobility of the first ray: a preliminary report. Foot Ankle Surg 2013;19(4):239–44.
37. Cottom JM, Rigby RB. Biomechanical comparison of a locking plate with intraplate compression screw versus locking plate with plantar interfragmentary screw for Lapidus arthrodesis: a cadaveric study. J Foot Ankle Surg 2013;52(3):339–42.
38. Cottom JM, Baker JS. Comparison of locking plate with interfragmentary screw versus plantarly applied anatomic locking plate for Lapidus arthrodesis: a biomechanical cadaveric study. Foot Ankle Spec 2017;10(3):227–31.
39. Aiyer A, Russell NA, Pelletier MH, et al. The impact of nitinol staples on the compressive forces, contact area, and mechanical properties in comparison to a claw plate and crossed screws for the first tarsometatarsal arthrodesis. Foot Ankle Spec 2016;9(3):232–40.
40. Feilmeier M, Dayton P, Kauwe M, et al. Comparison of transverse and coronal plane stability at the first tarsal-metatarsal joint with multiple screw orientations. Foot Ankle Spec 2017;10(2):104–8.

Intraoperative and Postoperative Evaluation of Hallux Valgus Correction
What Is Important?

Roberto Zambelli, MD[a],*, Daniel Baumfeld, MD, PhD[b,1]

KEYWORDS

- Hallux valgus • Triplane correction • Lapidus • Scarf • Bunion • Complications

KEY POINTS

- Hallux valgus is a triplane deformity and all planes should be understood and corrected for a good result.
- Preoperative evaluation is essential to determine the parameters to be corrected.
- Intraoperative fluoroscopy and perioperative clinical evaluation are reliable tools to be used during surgery.
- Special care in the postoperative period also can improve the final results.

INTRODUCTION

The hallux valgus (HA) is one of the most challenging foot and ankle deformities to correct. Clinicians recently have gained a better understanding of the preoperative evaluation based on specific parameters, and the main purpose is to find objective measurements that help understand the deformity and choose the correct way to achieve a well-aligned first ray, a harmonious forefoot, and a durable correction.

The concept of the metatarsus primus varus, valgus alignment of the hallux, hypermobility of the tarsometatarsal (TMT) joint,[1,2] and other different factors related to the HA deformity are well known, but all of them consider only a uniplanar evaluation of a multiplanar deformity. The actual concept is to consider the HA as a triplane deformity, and the parameters in (1) transverse, (2) sagittal, and (3) frontal planes must be considered.[3,4] Unsatisfactory results can be avoided if the correction includes all the 3 components, especially the derotation of the frontal plane.[4,5]

[a] Mater Dei Healthcare Network, Belo Horizonte, Minas Gerais, Brazil; [b] Federal University of Minas Gerais – UFMG, Felício Rocho Hospital, Belo Horizonte, Minas Gerais, Brazil
[1] Engenheiro Albert Scharle st 30/701, Belo Horizonte, Minas Gerais 30380-3070, Brazil.
* Corresponding author. Rua Ouro Preto 1016/405, Santo Agostinho, Belo Horizonte, Minas Gerais 30170-041, Brazil.
E-mail address: zambelliortop@gmail.com
Twitter: @drzambelli (R.Z.)

Foot Ankle Clin N Am 25 (2020) 127–139
https://doi.org/10.1016/j.fcl.2019.10.007
1083-7515/20/© 2019 Elsevier Inc. All rights reserved.

Foot and ankle surgeons can face difficulties during the surgery, which can lead to an unsatisfactory result. The under-correction and recurrence of the deformity are the most fearsome complications for the surgeons, and the search for tools and bony landmarks to avoid them has been an impetus in refining surgical technique. Most of these parameters are radiographic, as the HA angle, intermetatarsal angle (IMA), tibial sesamoid position (TSP),[1] and lateral edge of the first metatarsal head.[6]

The HA angle and IMA are traditional angles measured in a preoperative evaluation of a bunion deformity and also are reliable to determine the magnitude of the deformity in a weight-bearing anteroposterior (AP) radiograph.[7–9] Using only these 2 parameters, however, the HA is evaluated only in a 2-dimensional fashion, lacking the ability to address the coronal rotation of the first metatarsal.

The TSP and the roundness of the lateral edge of first metatarsal head are critical to understanding the frontal plane rotation. In contrast with the initial assumption, that sesamoids were just subluxated from their groove in a valgus deformity of the hallux, some investigators recently concluded that the sesamoid complex remains almost in its position whereas the metatarsal head drifts medially off its anchorage to the sesamoids, and the radiographic appearance of subluxation is the result of the medial deviation and also the rotation of the first metatarsal in frontal plane.[4,10–12] Considering these data, the radiographic appearance of the sesamoids is a consequence of the multiplane metatarsal deformity and not only changes in the sesamoid position.[4] The distance between the tibial sesamoid and the second metatarsal does not change in the preoperative and postoperative evaluations of the HA correction.[10,13]

The second key point to understanding the frontal plane rotation is the roundness of the lateral edge of the metatarsal head in patients with HA deformities. In a foot with an HA, the lateral and plantar aspects of the metatarsal head create a rounded appearance as the metatarsal assumes a pronated position, driving the great toe to valgus,[4,6,11,12,14–16] and its relationship with the deformity is statistically significant compared with normal feet.[6] Therefore, because the metatarsal head is an imperfect sphere, any change in its rotation results in corresponding clinical and radiographic changes in the direction and profile of the articular surface.[15]

The aim of this article is to discuss potential issues intraoperatively and postoperatively to evaluate the quality of the correction and to prevent recurrence during the HA correction.

PATIENT ASSESSMENT
Clinical Assessment

Patients should be initially evaluated in a standing position to address the magnitude of the hallux deformity and the possible associated injuries in the lesser toes, midfoot, and hindfoot.[1]

Moreover, surgeons should be aware of the mobility of the foot, especially the first metatarsophalangeal (MTP) and first TMT,[2,17,18] asymmetric hindfoot valgus,[19] gastrocnemius complex tightness,[20] and neurologic syndromes, which may affect treatment choice.

Radiographical Assessment

Clinicians should evaluate the deformity in more than 1 plane. Weight-bearing imaging of the forefoot and hindfoot is necessary. The sesamoid position is evaluated using both AP and tangential views. On the AP, the position of the sesamoid complex is measured by relating the medial sesamoid to the metatarsal axis,[21] grading in 7° of medial sesamoid position, considering displaced the medial sesamoid graded as V or more (**Fig. 1**).[22]

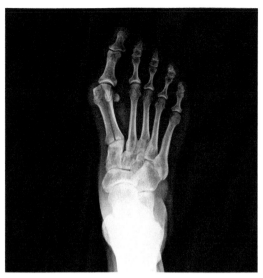

Fig. 1. Radiography showing the axis of the metatarsal bone and the medial sesamoid positioned lateral to the line.

Radiographical assessment of the sesamoid position on the tangential or axial view, as described by Talbot and Saltzman,[23] is considered a more reliable way to estimate the sesamoid malposition.[23] The sesamoids are considered reduced if the medial sesamoid is entirely medial to the midcristal line and unreduced if it is in any other position (**Fig. 2**).

The angle to be corrected (**Fig. 3**) is another radiographical measurement based on the rationale that the sesamoid complex remains in its position while the first metatarsal deviates medially in the HA deformity.[24] This angle has shown great interobserver correlation and is better than IMA to stratify patients to choose the ideal surgical technique.

The lateral edge of the first metatarsal head is classified in 3 groups: angular (type A), round (type R), or intermediate (type I). Surgeons must be concerned mostly with the round shape preoperatively; this is an important parameter to be corrected during surgery[6] (**Fig. 4**).

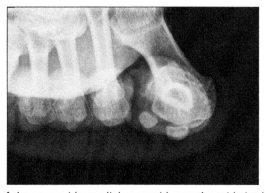

Fig. 2. Axial view of the sesamoids: medial sesamoid over the midcristal line.

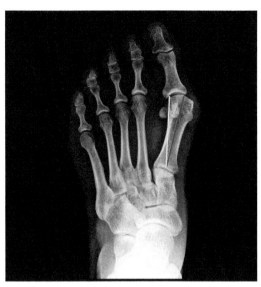

Fig. 3. Angle to be corrected: the red line is the axis of the first metatarsal and the yellow line is in the same starting point of the metatarsal axis through the middle of the sesamoid complex.

INTRAOPERATIVE EVALUATION

Intraoperative fluoroscopy is a reliable technique to be used during HA surgery and may help surgeons identify these parameters, cited previously, to correct and support a more accurate correction of the deformity.[25]

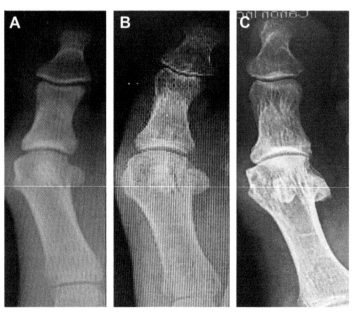

Fig. 4. Roundness of the lateral edge of the first metatarsal head. (A) Angular (type A); (B) round (type R); and (C) intermediate (type I).

Sesamoids

During the progression of HA, the metatarsal head deviates medially and pronates, while the sesamoid complex remains stable, held by the adductor tendon. Malreduction of the sesamoids increases the risk for recurrent deformity.[1]

To achieve a proper sesamoid correction in AP fluoroscopy view, the metatarsal head should be brought back to a more anatomic position, bringing the sesamoid with it, and not the opposite. The concept of pulling the sesamoid more medially or try to rely on soft tissue repositioning procedures, such as capsulorrhaphy and tendon releases, may not correct this complex deformity.[4,13] Relying only on the lateral soft tissue release and medial soft tissue plication as the main interventions to reorient the sesamoids position without the correction of the frontal plane rotation probably will fail, once the sesamoids begin to return their anatomic position in their grooves, which are still pronated.[14] Any unsatisfactory result in achieving this correction probably will lead to recurrence or misalignment.

The fluoroscopy AP and tangential views, as well as a direct observation of the medial sesamoid position, are crucial in this evaluation. Once the metatarsal osteotomy is performed, the surgeon should take care not to overcorrect the sesamoid malposition through the metatarsal osteotomy. In the fluoroscopy AP view, the medial border of the medial sesamoid cannot transpose the medial cortex of the first metatarsal; this could lead to an iatrogenic hallux varus.

Lateral Edge of First Metatarsal Head

The postoperative shape of the metatarsal head after an HA surgery has been linked with the recurrence of the deformity. The presence of a positive round sign on an intraoperative radiograph, even as intraoperative weight-bearing radiographs cannot be obtained properly, may suggest that pronation of the first metatarsal still remains and should be corrected, to lower the chances of recurrence.[6] Also, a direct visualization of the position of the metatarsal head and its relationship with the proximal phalanx base and the correction of the hallux position after the metatarsal osteotomy help the surgeon understand if the rotation was correct.

How to Control the Correction During Surgery?

Clinical evaluation and fluoroscopy images help surgeons during the operation time. Some techniques, however, do not allow triplane deformity correction. The proximal or extended procedures (osteotomies or arthrodesis) have higher ability to correct the frontal plane rotation associated with HA.[15,26,27] The authors consider the scarf osteotomy and the Lapidus procedures the most reliable techniques to address the parameter corrections, described previously.

Correction with scarf osteotomy

The scarf procedure is a versatile osteotomy. The length of the first metatarsal can be elongated, shortened, or maintained in the same position; the metatarsal, also can be plantar flexed, dorsiflexed or even rotated. To corrected all angular parameters related to HA deformity and first metatarsal malposition a preoperative plain must be accomplished.

The surgery is performed with traditional medial access to the first metatarsal and the first MTP. The inclination of the transverse cut determines the frontal plane correction (plantarflexion/dorsiflexion) of the first metatarsal. Later on, the 2 perpendicular cuts in the metatarsal, 1 dorsal and distal and another plantar and proximal, establish the 2 main fragments. A wedge of 5 mm in the plantar/distal fragment is performed to allow rotation and inclination of the main fragment that includes the metatarsal head (**Fig. 5**). If possible, a varus translation of the dorsal/proximal fragment should be performed to place the metatarsal-cuneiform joint in a position of greater instability (medial traction of the fragment). Rotation of the distal fragment also is performed to correct the coronal deformity (**Fig. 6**). The correction is performed under fluoroscopy with a provisional K-wire fixation and an acceptable correction is considered when the sesamoids are in a normal position (NP) under the metatarsal head and an angular shape of the lateral edge of the first metatarsal head is visualized (**Fig. 7**).

Definitive fixation is performed using 3 conventional screws with no compression, to allow the position to be maintained. The Akin osteotomy can be used concomitantly when the interphalangeal angle is increased. Then, a medial capsulorrhaphy and suture is performed traditionally.

Correction with Lapidus procedure

To assess intraoperative first MTP alignment, it is helpful to place K-wire in line on each side of the first tarsal metatarsal joint. A trick is to use the Hintermann spreader to guide the pin placement (**Fig. 8**), just to be sure that the K-wire are parallel. After the joint debridement and bone resection to correct the transverse and sagittal plane deformities, the pins should be used as a joystick to achieve rotational correction (**Fig. 9**). A provisional K-wire should be used to stabilize the fragments before the final fixation.

Under fluoroscopy guidance, the align position of sesamoids and the decrease of lateral round sign of the metatarsal head can be visualized and the definitive fixation can be performed.[14]

Maximizing IMA to stress the instability of TMT joint to prevent recurrence of the deformity is another option to use during the surgical intervention.[28–30] This rationale is used in both open and percutaneous procedures. This varus displacement of the proximal fragment can be done by pulling the fragment using Backhaus forceps[29]

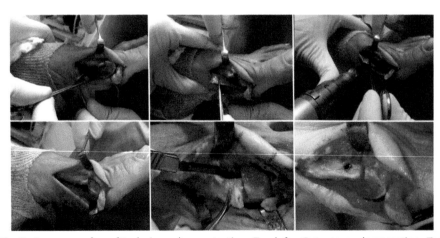

Fig. 5. Sequence of scarf technique demonstration. *Top left* – Osteotomy demarcation. *Top middle* – Two main fragments demonstration. *Top Right* – Proximal wedge resection of plantar distal fragment. *Bottom left* – Reposition the fragments to check possible correction. *Bottom middle* – Releasing the soft tissue adhesion of the dorsal proximal fragment. *Bottom right* – Fragments fixated in a proper position.

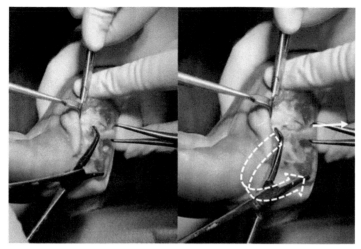

Fig. 6. Varus translation of the dorsal/proximal fragment (*solid arrow*). Rotation of the distal fragment (*square dot arrow*). *Left* – Two Backhaus forceps positioned to correct rotation and varus of the first metatarsal. *Right* – Varus translation of the dorsal/proximal fragment and rotation of the plantar/distal fragment.

or a 2.0 K-wire as a joystick, then pinning the first metatarsal to the second metatarsal, to hold the fragment while doing the corrective osteotomy on the metatarsal bone[30] (**Fig. 10**).

POSTOPERATIVE CARE

To allow a comfortable and safe postoperative period after an HA correction, surgeons must consider 4 main parameters: pain management, swelling control, safe walking with postoperative shoes, and alignment maintenance.

The literature demonstrates that a nerve block adjuvant to general anesthesia reduces postsurgical pain and improves functional outcomes in HA surgery. When comparing patients who had and had not nerve block, those with nerve block walk earlier, demonstrate an improved visual analog scale score, and use less medication at home. For that reason, it is recommended to add a peripheral nerve block after the HA correction[31]

Edema control, safe walking, and alignment maintenance can be achieved using postoperative taping (**Fig. 11**). The literature has demonstrated no radiographic

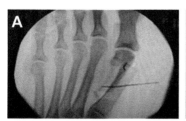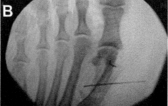

Fig. 7. Scarf osteotomy with fluoroscopy demonstration. (*A*) Insufficient correction; inclination was not corrected. (*B*) Correction of all 3 planes achieved.

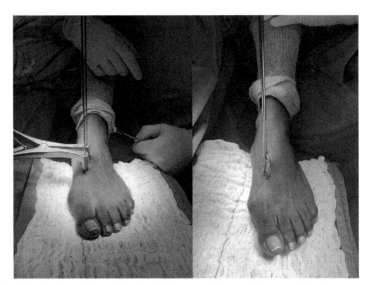

Fig. 8. Positioning the 2.0-mm K-wires in the medial cuneiform and first metatarsal using the Hintermann spreader (*left*) to ensure they are parallel (*right*).

benefit of postoperative dynamic immobilization after hallux correction[32]; however, the authors do not expect radiographic changing using the taping technique. The main objective is to provide a more comfortable and safer postoperative period. Dressings are changed every 10 days and remain for at least 6 weeks. They allow a controlled MTP joint mobilization, with no damage to the soft tissue, and an external stabilization of the metatarsal, to give the sensation of a stable forefoot. In a nonpublished data analysis, patients report more comfortable and safe walking then those who have not used the taping management.

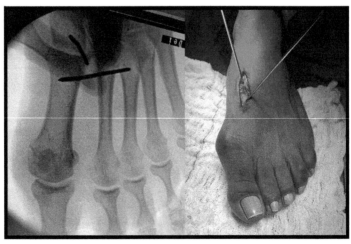

Fig. 9. Fluoroscopy image (*left*) and the clinical aspect (*right*) after the correction of the triplane deformity of the first ray.

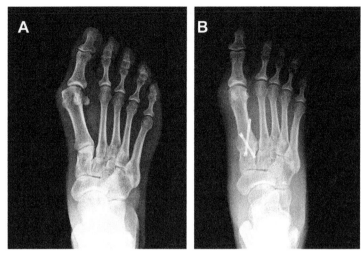

Fig. 10. Preoperative (*A*) and postoperative (*B*) images of a Lapidus correction.

DISCUSSION
Sesamoids

Esemenli and colleagues[33] assessed the relation between the reduction of the metatarsal head over the sesamoid complex and the correction of the distal osteotomy. They assessed the position of the medial sesamoid, which was considered displaced if the medial sesamoid was overlapping the midaxial line more than 50%. Twenty-three patients (30 feet) submitted to a distal oblique osteotomy were included, and they found, at 32 months of follow-up, that 20 had reduced and 10 had unreduced sesamoids. The reduced and unreduced groups were significantly different with respect to their preoperative HA angle and IMA, the average postoperative HA angle was 14.4° in the sesamoid reduced group and 23.6° in the sesamoid unreduced group (P<.0001). Moreover, the lateral displacement (DIS) of the metatarsal head was found to have a statistically significant role in reducing the sesamoids, with means of 8.5 mm in the reduced group and 4.1 mm in the unreduced group (P<.0005; 95% CI, 7.243–9.757).

Okuda and colleagues[22] also demonstrated the role of the sesamoid malposition after proximal crescentic osteotomy for treatment of HA in the recurrence of the

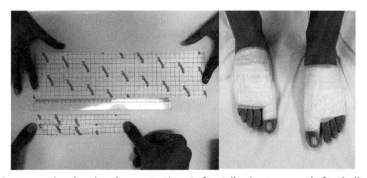

Fig. 11. Postoperative dressing demonstration. *Left* – Adhesive tape used after hallux valgus surgery. *Right* – Dynamic dressing in a bilateral Hallux valgus correction.

deformity. A case-control study with 43 patients (65 feet) in the operated group and 60 feet in the control group was conducted, used as a reference for the medial sesamoid position, stating that the NP is grade IV or less, according to Hardy and Clapham classification.[21] Patients were divided in 2 groups: the NP group and the DIS group, with the sesamoid position graded as V or more. The HA angle in the NP group varied from a mean of 10.8° at the early follow-up to 12.0° at the latest follow-up (P = .0843), whereas in the DIS group it varied from 15.0° to 19.5° (P = .0082). In terms of recurrence, 13% of the feet included in the NP group and 59% of the DIS group presented with recurrence.

In a study to evaluate risk factors for recurrence of HA, Shibuya and colleagues[34] reported that the sesamoid position after surgery is the only significant factor related to recurrence. Their analysis showed a postoperative TSP greater than 4 increases the recurrence 3-fold (odds ratio [OR] 3.4; 95% CI, 1.54 to 7.66), with a recurrence rate of 51%, and also a stronger association if TSP is greater than 5 (OR 4.4; 95% CI, 1.59–12.69), with a recurrence rate of 60%.

Achieving the goal of reducing the sesamoids under the metatarsal head, however, is not an easy task. A learning curve and the ability to understand the complexity of the deformity and also to perceive the tridimensional change of each corrective osteotomy are mandatory. Seng and colleagues[35] evaluated the quality of the reduction of the sesamoids among 65 consecutive patients who had undergone a scarf osteotomy after 6 months of surgery. The patients were allocated in 3 groups according to the date of surgery, with the first 24 consecutive patients in group 1, the next 24 in group 2, and the last 23 in group 3. A significant difference was found in the median postoperative sesamoid position of groups 1 and 2 (P = .027) and between groups 1 and 3 (P = .001).

Based on the findings discussed previously, it is absolutely necessary to obtain intraoperative confirmation that the sesamoids are reduced under the first metatarsal head after surgical correction of HA deformity to prevent recurrence.

Lateral Edge of Fist Metatarsal Head

The first to discuss this relationship was Okuda and colleagues[6] in a retrospective study where they compared the shape of the head between women with moderate to severe deformities and normal controls, matched by age and sex, preoperatively. They observed that the prevalence of type R–shaped metatarsal head in the HA group before surgery was significantly higher than in the control group (P<.0001), suggesting that there is a strong relationship between the shape of the metatarsal head and the occurrence of HA. Regarding recurrence, the authors found that a positive round sign at the time of the early follow-up was associated with a greater risk of having recurrence of the HA deformity than a negative round sign—type A or type I—at the time of the early follow-up (OR 12.71; 95% CI, 3.2–50.36).

Other investigators also correlated the absence of the rounded sign on the curvature of the lateral cortical surface of the metatarsal head after surgery as a predictor of success of the intervention.[12,14,28] Okuda and colleagues[27] founded 11 positive rounded signs preoperatively and 11 negative rounded signs after surgery, in a group of 12 adolescents who underwent a proximal abduction-supination osteotomy of the first metatarsal at the most recent follow-up radiographs, concluding that these factors led to no recurrence in their patients.

SUMMARY

Recurrence and loss of correction are common complications after HA corrective surgery. Although many investigators have studied the risk factors associated with a suboptimal hallux position at the end of long-term follow-up, only a few have demonstrated which parameters should be analyzed preoperatively and how they should be evaluated intraoperatively during this deformity correction. The sesamoid position and the shape of the metatarsal head are actually the most reliable to consider. The authors have demonstrated techniques that could achieve this objective as well as the postoperative management to perform a safe and durable correction.

DISCLOSURE

R. Zambelli has nothing to disclose. D. Baumfeld is consultant/speaker—Arthrex, MSD (Merck Sharp Dome).

REFERENCES

1. Coughlin MJ. Instructional course lectures, The American Academy of Orthopaedic Surgeons - Hallux Valgus. J Bone Joint Surg Am 1996;78(6):932–66.
2. Coughlin MJ, Jones CP. Hallux valgus and first ray mobility. A prospective study. J Bone Joint Surg Am 2007;89(9):1887–98.
3. Scranton PE, Rutkowski R. Anatomic variations in the first ray: Part I. Anatomic aspects related to bunion surgery. Clin Orthop Relat Res 1980;(151):244–55.
4. Dayton P, Feilmeier M, Hirschi J, et al. Observed changes in radiographic measurements of the first ray after frontal plane rotation of the first metatarsal in a cadaveric foot model. J Foot Ankle Surg 2014;53(3):274–8.
5. Welck MJ, Al-Khudairi N. Imaging of hallux valgus: how to approach the deformity. Foot Ankle Clin 2018;23(2):183–92.
6. Okuda R, Kinoshita M, Yasuda T, et al. The shape of the lateral edge of the first metatarsal head as a risk factor for recurrence of hallux valgus. J Bone Joint Surg Am 2007;89(10):2163–72.
7. Coughlin MJ, Saltzman CL, Nunley JA. Angular measurements in the evaluation of hallux valgus deformities: a report of the ad hoc committee of the American Orthopaedic Foot & Ankle Society on angular measurements. Foot Ankle Int 2002; 23(1):68–74.
8. Coughlin MJ, Freund E. Roger A. Mann Award. The reliability of angular measurements in hallux valgus deformities. Foot Ankle Int 2001;22(5):369–79.
9. Lee KM, Ahn S, Chung CY, et al. Reliability and relationship of radiographic measurements in hallux valgus. Clin Orthop Relat Res 2012;470(9):2613–21.
10. Ramdass R, Meyr AJ. The multiplanar effect of first metatarsal osteotomy on sesamoid position. J Foot Ankle Surg 2010;49(1):63–7.
11. Dayton P, Feilmeier M, Kauwe M, et al. Observed changes in radiographic measurements of the first ray after frontal and transverse plane rotation of the hallux: does the hallux drive the metatarsal in a bunion deformity? J Foot Ankle Surg 2014;53(5):584–7.
12. Dayton P, Feilmeier M. Comparison of tibial sesamoid position on anteroposterior and axial radiographs before and after triplane tarsal metatarsal joint arthrodesis. J Foot Ankle Surg 2017;56(5):1041–6.
13. Choi YR, Lee S-J, Kim JH, et al. Effect of metatarsal osteotomy and open lateral soft tissue procedure on sesamoid position: radiological assessment. J Orthop Surg Res 2018;13(1):11.

14. Dayton P, Kauwe M, Feilmeier M. Is our current paradigm for evaluation and management of the bunion deformity flawed? A discussion of procedure philosophy relative to anatomy. J Foot Ankle Surg 2015;54(1):102–11.

15. Dayton P, Feilmeier M, Kauwe M, et al. Relationship of frontal plane rotation of first metatarsal to proximal articular set angle and hallux alignment in patients undergoing tarsometatarsal arthrodesis for hallux abducto valgus: a case series and critical review of the literature. J Foot Ankle Surg 2013;52(3):348–54.

16. Dayton P, Kauwe M, DiDomenico L, et al. Quantitative analysis of the degree of frontal rotation required to anatomically align the first metatarsal phalangeal joint during modified tarsal-metatarsal arthrodesis without capsular balancing. J Foot Ankle Surg 2016;55(2):220–5.

17. Shibuya N, Roukis TS, Jupiter DC. Mobility of the first ray in patients with or without hallux valgus deformity: systematic review and meta-analysis. J Foot Ankle Surg 2017;56(5):1070–5.

18. Steinberg N, Finestone A, Noff M, et al. Relationship between lower extremity alignment and hallux valgus in women. Foot Ankle Int 2013;34(6):824–31.

19. King DM, Toolan BC. Associated deformities and hypermobility in hallux valgus: an investigation with weightbearing radiographs. Foot Ankle Int 2004;25(4):251–5.

20. Barouk LS. The effect of gastrocnemius tightness on the pathogenesis of juvenile hallux valgus: a preliminary study. Foot Ankle Clin 2014;19(4):807–22.

21. Hardy RH, Clapham JCR. Observations on hallux valgus; based on a controlled series. J Bone Joint Surg Br 1951;33-B(3):376–91.

22. Okuda R, Kinoshita M, Yasuda T, et al. Postoperative incomplete reduction of the sesamoids as a risk factor for recurrence of hallux valgus. J Bone Joint Surg Am 2009;91(7):1637–45.

23. Talbot KD, Saltzman CL. Assessing sesamoid subluxation: how good is the AP radiograph? Foot Ankle Int 1998;19(8):547–54.

24. Ortiz C, Wagner P, Vela O, et al. "Angle to be corrected" in preoperative evaluation for hallux valgus Surgery. Foot Ankle Int 2015;37(2):172–7.

25. Elliot RR, Saxby TS, Whitehouse SL. Intraoperative imaging in hallux valgus surgery. Foot Ankle Surg 2012;18(1):19–21.

26. Huang EH, Charlton TP, Ajayi S, et al. Effect of various hallux valgus reconstruction on sesamoid location: a radiographic study. Foot Ankle Int 2013;34(1):99–103.

27. Okuda R, Yasuda T, Jotoku T, et al. Proximal abduction–supination osteotomy of the first metatarsal for adolescent hallux valgus: a preliminary report. J Orthop Sci 2013;18(3):419–25.

28. Yasuda T, Okuda R, Jotoku T, et al. Proximal supination osteotomy of the first metatarsal for hallux valgus. Foot Ankle Int 2015;36(6):696–704.

29. Prudente HM, Baumfeld DS, Baumfeld TS, et al. Increased intermetatarsal angle of the proximal fragment after modified scarf osteotomy. Sci J Foot Ankle 2018;12(3):1–6.

30. Vernois J, Redfern DJ. Percutaneous surgery for severe hallux valgus. Foot Ankle Clin 2016;21(3):479–93.

31. Kir MC, Kir G. Ankle nerve block adjuvant to general anesthesia reduces postsurgical pain and improves functional outcomes in hallux valgus surgery. Med Princ Pract 2018;27(3):236–40.

32. Ponzio DY, Pedowitz DI, Verma K, et al. Radiographic outcomes of postoperative taping following hallux valgus correction. Foot Ankle Int 2015;36(7):820–6.

33. Esemenli T, Yildirim Y, Bezer M. Lateral shifting of the first metatarsal head in hallux valgus surgery: effect on sesamoid reduction. Foot Ankle Int 2003; 24(12):922–6.
34. Shibuya N, Kyprios EM, Panchani PN, et al. Factors associated with early loss of hallux valgus correction. J Foot Ankle Surg 2018;57(2):236–40.
35. Seng C, Chunyin Ho D, Chong KW. Restoring sesamoid position in scarf osteotomy: a learning curve. J Foot Ankle Surg 2015;54(6):1089–92.

Postoperative Considerations in the Management of Hallux Valgus

William A. Hester III, MD[a], David I. Pedowitz, MS, MD[b],*

KEYWORDS

- Hallux valgus • Postoperative management • Patient expectations
- Pain management • Weight bearing • Immobilization • Return to activity

KEY POINTS

- It is important to set patient expectations prior to hallux valgus correction surgery.
- Postoperative pain management is achieved with a multimodal approach using regional blocks, minimal narcotics, nonsteroidal anti-inflammatory drugs, and other modalities as necessary.
- Immobilization and weight bearing activities can be progressed quicker than historically taught.

INTRODUCTION

As surgeries to treat hallux valgus have evolved over the decades, postoperative treatment regimens have largely changed as well. Although many of these are not standardized, there are myriad postoperative protocols that have evolved to minimize morbidity and increase patient satisfaction. This chapter focuses on current concepts of the postoperative period, including pain management, immobilization, weight bearing restrictions, physical therapy, and return to activity.

MANAGING EXPECTATIONS

Surgeons frequently base their idea of a successful surgery on pain reduction, postoperative radiographs, and clinical appearance. Although these variables are important, patients often judge the success of surgeries based on other criteria. The authors suggest that when approaching a patient with a hallux valgus deformity, managing patient expectations is equally as important as achieving radiographic and clinical correction of deformity.

[a] Sidney Kimmel Medical College, Thomas Jefferson University, The Rothman Institute, 925 Chestnut Street, 5th Floor, Philadelphia, PA 19107, USA; [b] Foot & Ankle Fellowship, Sidney Kimmel Medical College, Thomas Jefferson University, The Rothman Institute, 925 Chestnut Street, 5th Floor, Philadelphia, PA 19107, USA
* Corresponding author.
E-mail address: David.Pedowitz@rothmanortho.com

Foot Ankle Clin N Am 25 (2020) 141–150
https://doi.org/10.1016/j.fcl.2019.11.002
1083-7515/20/© 2019 Elsevier Inc. All rights reserved.

Managing patient expectations requires a frank conversation preoperatively to set out realistic milestones and an understanding of what is and what is not achievable. Hallux valgus correction is painful and inconvenient, and it has a lengthy recovery period that patients largely minimize in their own minds. Additionally, the emotional components of desired shoe wear, sports participation, and the degree of cosmetic deformity correction should not be underestimated. For this surgery to be successful, patients need time to digest the entire scope of the surgery and its recovery.

Patients also need to be informed that pain reduction is the primary goal of surgery, with deformity correction as a secondary goal. For many patients, this order is reversed in their minds. If patients understand that surgeons are treating their painful bunion first and deformity second, patient and physician postoperative expectations may become more aligned.

In the authors' experience, patients frequently expect that bunion surgery is a simple operation that involves a quick recovery. Many surgeons may agree with this, but their perceptions compared with patients' perceptions of what a quick recovery is may be quite different. Patients must understand that most physicians have postoperative dressing requirements and weight-bearing restrictions that must be followed for adequate bone and wound healing. Patients should also understand that their foot will continue to swell for at least several months after their wounds heal. Although these discomforts are temporary, they are inconvenient and interfere significantly with shoe wear. Surgeons should discuss with patients that shoes are like gloves, in that they require a precise fit to be comfortable. Patients with a swollen foot have pain and difficulty with many shoes once they are allowed to return to regular shoe wear. They should be counseled that swelling is normal, and it can take up to 6 months to return to their desired shoe wear comfortably.

POSTOPERATIVE PAIN MANAGEMENT

Just as patients expect hallux valgus correction to be a simple surgery, many times they expect minimal to no pain in the recovery period. Surgeons should educate their patients that there will be some pain after surgery but that the surgeons will help them to make it safely manageable. Seymour and colleagues[1] recommend, "To help our patients get comfortable, we need to develop, support, and champion comprehensive approaches to pain relief." This includes not only medications but also these discussions. Screening for depression and poor coping skills can help determine which patients will seek more opiate therapy. This can be as simple as asking questions, such as, "How did you cope with pain after your last surgery?" or "Have you ever been treated for depression?"[1] Although legislation in many states now restricts postoperative narcotic prescriptions, preoperatively setting strict limits of how many pills patients are provided with after surgery can be a helpful tactic to decrease reliance on opioids. These limits help patients set their expectations for how much pain medication they should need after surgery. It also indicates that there is not an endless supply of prescriptions coming from the surgeon. Patients with depression have been shown to be less satisfied with their postoperative pain control. Shakked and colleagues found that patients with depression also had less pain according to their visual analog scale (VAS) pain scores,[2] highlighting the difficulty with obtaining patient satisfaction in those carrying a depression diagnosis.

Regional Blocks

Postoperative pain management has gained more attention now as physicians deal with the current opioid crisis. To this end, gaining adequate control of pain from surgery must be balanced with preventing narcotic abuse and addiction. Multimodal pain regimens focus on this goal by using several methods to control surgical pain. Studies are now focusing on fine-tuning pain control and safety. Performing an ankle block with local infiltration in patients undergoing general anesthesia has been shown to have shorter hospital stays and less need for narcotic pain medicine in the postoperative period.[3] Another trial found that if a local infiltration block is to be performed, although perhaps inconvenient, it seems more effective if done after tourniquet inflation.[4] Schipper and colleagues[5] demonstrated better immediate postoperative pain control and decreased opioid requirements with a popliteal fossa block compared with an ankle block in forefoot surgeries. Regional anesthesia increasingly is used as an adjunct for perioperative pain management in an effort to decrease the amount of narcotics needed postoperatively.[6,7] Ambrosoli and colleagues[8] determined the optimal placement of a popliteal nerve catheter tip to minimize long-term complications and achieve the best perioperative pain control.

Local anesthetic injections in and around the wound also have been studied. Liposomal bupivacaine has been popular in the recent literature. Robbins and colleagues[9] studied its use in forefoot surgery comparing ankle block alone to ankle block with wound infiltration with liposomal bupivacaine. Their numbers were small, but the investigators found that the liposomal bupivacaine group had decreased oral narcotic use in the first 2 days, fewer narcotic refills, and longer times to the first refill if needed. They also found a trend toward decreased pain scores in the first 4 postoperative days. Although cost for this medication remains an issue for many centers, its effectiveness and ease of administration should not be overlooked and it should still be considered an option for surgeons looking to prevent postoperative pain at the surgical site.

Narcotic Use

After regional blocks stop working, patients rely on oral medications for adequate pain control. Historically, this was achieved with opioid and opioid-like medications. There are no well-established guidelines to narcotic prescriptions in the postoperative period. Just as each surgeon applies a different postoperative dressing, surveys have found no consensus in narcotic prescribing principles.[10,11] Finney and colleagues[12] found a rate of approximately 6% persistent opioid use (>91 days) after hallux valgus surgery in opioid-naïve patients. The authors found persistent opioid used was associated with equivalent doses of greater than 45 tablets of oxycodone, 5 mg; patients who filled a narcotic pain prescription within 30 days prior to surgery; geographic regions outside the Northeast United States; and certain mental health conditions. Furthermore, Rogero and colleagues[13] found no difference between opioid requirements when differentiated on which procedure was performed for hallux valgus correction. In this study, chevron osteotomies, proximal osteotomies (Ludloff and scarf), soft tissue–only procedures with or without a first proximal phalanx osteotomy (modified McBride and Akin), and first metatarsophalangeal arthrodeses were compared. The investigators found a low rate of persistent opioid use, but patients with preexisting pain conditions were excluded from this study. These 2 studies together imply that physicians should be having discussions about pain medication use during the preoperative appointment. Proper counseling and awareness of risk factors may help decrease the rate of persistent opioid use after hallux valgus correction.

As the nation has become aware of the opioid crisis, the responsibility of the prescriber has increased. It has been shown that patients taking opioids longer than 12 weeks postoperatively demonstrated a 50% risk of continuing them at 5 years.[14]

Physicians strive to make patients more comfortable by treating their pain. Most physicians agree that it is inappropriate for patients to be on opioids for 12 weeks after bunion surgery, but if the prescriber is not cognizant of weaning patients from opioids, this situation can easily happen.

Role of Other Agents

Other medications have been studied as part of a multimodal pain regimen to further decrease the narcotics required for adequate pain control. Nonsteroidal anti-inflammatory drugs (NSAIDs) also have been used as an adjunct for postoperative pain control. There is concern that they may interfere with bone growth after osteotomies or arthrodesis procedures because delayed bone healing has been shown in animal models and some in vitro studies.[15–18] Hassan and Karlock[19] performed a retrospective study looking for an association between NSAID use and nonunion in foot and ankle surgery requiring bony work. Specifically, they looked at patients using ketorolac and ibuprofen in the postoperative period for 2 weeks or less. The investigators found no association between NSAID use and nonunion in their cohort. They recommend using these drugs for a short time period (up to 2 weeks) for postoperative pain control. A meta-analysis showed that NSAIDs used for a short duration or in low doses did not increase risk of delayed union/nonunion for fracture, osteotomy, or arthrodesis.[16] This review did demonstrate increased delayed union and nonunion rates with long-term NSAID use. In a small study, oral glucocorticoids administered in the postanesthesia care unit and 24 hours later at home showed promising results in decreasing postoperative opioid use for patients undergoing first metatarsal osteotomy.[20] Two systematic reviews have shown that high-dose steroids administered in a short time period do not cause an increase in the rate of wound problems or postoperative infections.[21,22] These results reveal that long-held beliefs about NSAIDs and glucocorticoids in the postoperative period may not be as harmful to orthopedic surgery in the foot and ankle as was once thought.

Authors' Preference

At the authors' institution, patients are extensively counseled about the current opioid crisis, current trends in prescribing pain medication, statewide legislation, and the surgeon's preferred protocol. Unless a sensitivity has been documented previously, patients are given 20 tablets of oxycodone/acetaminophen (5 mg / 325 mg) for pain and 10 tablets of ondansetron (4 mg) for nausea. No refills are provided. Should additional analgesia be needed, patients are given ketorolac (10 mg) as needed. Each patient is administered an ankle block with 0.5% bupivacaine (30 mL) and 1% lidocaine (10 mL) immediately prior to surgery after induction of anesthesia. The authors have found this a safe and effective protocol, which has resulted in a high patient satisfaction with postoperative pain management.

ROLE OF IMMOBILIZATION

Two primary concerns postoperatively for every surgeon are maintaining correction of deformity and ensuring adequate bony and soft tissue healing. To this end, a variety of strategies have been developed and many vary considerably. The essential variables are the degree and timing of weight bearing and the use or need for strapping devices. Historically, patients were made non–weight bearing after bunion surgery. With the advent of more stable and reliable permanent internal fixation, safer and early weight bearing in less immobilization may be achieved.

The classic teaching states that the operative foot should be immobilized for a period of 6 weeks to 8 weeks using either a short leg cast, boot, or heel–weight bearing postoperative shoe.[23–25] During this time period, the recommendation has been taping of the toe with a spica-like dressing to hold the toe in neutral or slight varus/valgus position. Pentikäinen and colleagues[26] compared soft cast versus elastic bandage for postoperative care after distal chevron osteotomies and found no difference in American Orthopaedic Foot and Ankle Society (AOFAS) scores or hallux valgus recurrence at final follow-up. They recommended, therefore, elastic bandage only. Basile and colleagues[27] compared patients who were treated with a first metatarsal–medial cuneiform (MTC) arthrodesis and placed into a short leg cast and non–weight bearing versus boot with immediate partial weight bearing through the heel. Those patients treated with immediate partial weight bearing had an additional Kirschner wire across the fusion site. At final follow-up, no nonunions or malunions were identified, and there was no difference in first intermetatarsal angle and first ray elevation between groups. Kazzaz and Singh[28] evaluated a cohort of patients undergoing MTC arthrodesis and treated postoperatively with a wedge shoe instead of a cast. They found no nonunions in their group of 27 patients.

The spica taping procedure requires retaping the toe weekly after removing the initial compressive dressing. This process typically involves weekly office visits for up to 8 weeks. Ponzio and colleagues looked at spica taping versus foam toe spacer use after Ludloff osteotomy with modified McBride distal soft tissue release.[29] The initial dressings were left on for 2 weeks. Patients then received weekly spica taping for 6 weeks or a large foam toe spacer. There were no clinically significant differences in lasting deformity correction between the 2 groups, suggesting that postoperative toe taping may not be necessary.

Authors' Preference

At the authors' institution all patients are placed in a bunion spica dressing postoperatively, which is changed 4 days to 5 days later for comfort. The dressing is removed at 2 weeks for suture removal and then only a toe spacer is used until the eighth postoperative week.

TIMING OF WEIGHT BEARING

Weight-bearing recommendations after hallux valgus correction remain anecdotal because no evidence-based published guidelines exist. The decision for weight bearing, therefore, remains diverse, with some surgeons allowing immediate weight bearing in a postoperative shoe. Other surgeons make patients non–weight bearing for 2 weeks and then allow weight bearing in a forefoot unloading shoe or a regular stiff-soled postoperative shoe until the eighth week. Partial weight-bearing recommendations generally are by physician preference. These recommendations are modified based on the procedure performed.

For distal soft tissue realignment or distal chevron osteotomy procedures, patients typically are allowed to weight bear as tolerated immediately or by 2 weeks in a heel-weight bearing postoperative shoe.[30–32] This continues for up to 6 weeks.[25,33] There is a paucity in the literature studying specific weight bearing protocols in these procedures.

Historically, patients who were treated with proximal osteotomies initially are placed in a below-knee cast, heel-weight bearing postoperative shoe, or boot, depending on the surgeon.[25,34,35] Liszka and Gadek[36] compared patients treated with a scarf osteotomy secured with fixation versus no fixation and allowed all groups to immediately weight bear as tolerated with a heel-bearing boot. They found comparable satisfactory results between the groups.[36] Patients treated with proximal opening wedge osteotomies have shown that it is safe to weight bear as tolerated in a heel-weight bearing shoe if the lateral cortex is maintained. If the lateral cortex is violated, non–weight bearing is recommended until radiographic union is demonstrated to avoid risk of nonunion.[37]

Traditionally, patients are kept non–weight bearing and immobilized in a cast for 6 weeks to 8 weeks after first MTC arthrodesis. Progressive weight bearing usually begins after 4 weeks to 6 weeks.[23–25] Early results of MTC arthrodesis reported a nonunion rate of 6.4% in patients who were kept non–weight bearing for 6 weeks to 10 weeks.[38] A level IV review looked at nonunion rates with early weight bearing after MTC arthrodesis.[39] Some investigators allowed weight bearing to begin at 2 weeks in a cast or cast boot; others started immediate weight bearing in a wedged shoe, short cast boot, or walking cast after arthrodesis. Specifically, this retrospective review looked at 443 arthrodeses and found a nonunion rate of approximately 3.6% with early weight bearing. Unfortunately, there was no comparative cohort in any of the studies that were reviewed. A multicenter study of 57 patients found a low incidence of symptomatic nonunions (1.6%) and recurrence (3.2%) after patients were allowed early (<2 weeks) full weight bearing when undergoing MTC arthrodesis.[40] The largest study looking at nonunion included 136 patients and allowed partial weight bearing in a cast boot at nearly 2 weeks postoperatively.[41] They report a nonunion rate of 2.21%. These results seem to imply that early, protected weight bearing after MTC arthrodesis does not increase nonunion rates.

Authors' Preference

At the authors' institution, patients are made heel-only weight bearing for transfers and are instructed to use crutches for 2 weeks. Afterward, patients are permitted to be weight bearing as tolerated in a stiff-soled postoperative shoe until the eighth week, at which point regular shoe wear is permitted.

ROLE OF PHYSICAL THERAPY

As immobilization has decreased, emphasis on postoperative early range-of-motion (ROM) exercises has increased. With distal procedures requiring minimal immobilization, the recommendation is to start active and passive ROM exercises as pain allows.[25] The literature on rehabilitation after hallux valgus correction is sparse. Schuh and colleagues[42] studied plantar pressure distribution in a group of patients who underwent correction with either a scarf osteotomy or distal chevron osteotomy and were treated with physical therapy. They were able to show a trend toward increased forces across the great toe and first metatarsal head regions compared with preoperative values. They also demonstrated increased AOFAS scores in both groups. It is difficult to draw definitive conclusions about physical therapy's role in the postoperative treatment course based on this study because their results did not reach statistical significance and there was no control group. There have been several studies on pedobarographic parameters after hallux valgus correction. These studies have shown that pressure along the first ray is decreased compared with preoperative values.[43–46] These data indicate that there may be a role for physical therapy to help better normalize gait patterns. More research is needed in this area to determine timing and duration of physical therapy as well as which exercises are beneficial.

Authors' Preference

The authors feel strongly that routine postoperative physical therapy is not necessary but should be used on a case-by-case basis because some patients (those with balance or presurgical gait dysfunction or additional gait-related comorbidities) may significantly benefit from its use.

RETURN TO ACTIVITY

Most patients are fully weight bearing without any immobilization by 10 weeks to 12 weeks postoperatively regardless of the corrective procedure performed. This is different from resuming driving and preoperative exercise levels. In a prospective study, Coetzee and Wickum[47] allowed patients to return to full activities at 3 months. They reported that 96% were able to return to their level of function prior to their bunion causing pain. The average age in their study was 41 years. MacMahon and colleagues[48] reviewed return to sporting activities in patients undergoing MTC arthrodesis for hallux valgus in patients ages 14 years to 49 years. They found that only 79% of these patients were able to return to their preoperative exercise level at final follow-up.

The authors' institution conducted a prospective study on brake response time after right-sided first metatarsal osteotomy for hallux valgus correction.[49] The results demonstrated that 85% of patients were safe to drive at 6 weeks and 100% were safe to drive at 8 weeks. Those who were not ready at 6 weeks had higher VAS scores and lower metatarsophalangeal joint ROM and reported that they were not comfortable with driving. Holt and colleagues[50] performed a similar study and demonstrated that only 25% were safe to drive at 2 weeks, but 100% of their cohort were safe to drive at 6 weeks. Some patients feel that they are safe to drive with a postoperative shoe. Brake reaction time was studied in Austria, where the investigators found significantly impaired times compared with preoperative values.[51] From these results, it seems that driving is safe 6 weeks to 8 weeks postoperatively if a patient is allowed out of all immobilization. Patients also should demonstrate low VAS scores and feel that they are mentally prepared to stop quickly if they need to. The authors routinely recommend that patients go to an empty parking lot and practice driving in a controlled environment. The authors instruct them to attempt several quick stops to make sure this is a pain-free procedure.

DISCLOSURE

Nothing to disclose.

REFERENCES

1. Seymour RB, Ring D, Higgins T, et al. Leading the way to solutions to the opioid epidemic: AOA critical issues. J Bone Joint Surg Am 2017;99(21):e113.
2. Shakked R, McDonald E, Sutton R, et al. Influence of depressive symptoms on hallux valgus surgical outcomes. Foot Ankle Int 2018;39(7):795–800.
3. Kir MC, Kir G. Ankle nerve block adjuvant to general anesthesia reduces postsurgical pain and improves functional outcomes in hallux valgus surgery. Med Princ Pract 2018;27(3):236–40.
4. Singh VK, Ridgers S, Sott AH. Ankle block in forefoot reconstruction before or after inflation of tourniquet–Does timing matter? Foot Ankle Surg 2013;19(1):15–7.
5. Schipper ON, Hunt KJ, Anderson RB, et al. Ankle block vs single-shot popliteal fossa block as primary anesthesia for forefoot operative procedures: prospective, randomized comparison. Foot Ankle Int 2017;38(11):1188–91.
6. Gupta A, Kumar K, Roberts MM, et al. Pain management after outpatient foot and ankle surgery. Foot Ankle Int 2018;39(2):149–54.

7. Choi GW, Kim HJ, Kim TS, et al. Comparison of the modified McBride procedure and the distal chevron osteotomy for mild to moderate hallux valgus. J Foot Ankle Surg 2016;55(4):808–11.

8. Ambrosoli AL, Guzzetti L, Chiaranda M, et al. A randomised controlled trial comparing two popliteal nerve catheter tip positions for postoperative analgesia after day-case hallux valgus repair. Anaesthesia 2016;71(11):1317–23.

9. Robbins J, Green CL, Parekh SG. Liposomal bupivacaine in forefoot surgery. Foot Ankle Int 2015;36(5):503–7.

10. Wunsch H, Wijeysundera DN, Passarella MA, et al. Opioids prescribed after low-risk surgical procedures in the United States, 2004-2012. JAMA 2016;315(15): 1654–7.

11. Sabatino MJ, Kunkel ST, Ramkumar DB, et al. Excess opioid medication and variation in prescribing patterns following common orthopaedic procedures. J Bone Joint Surg Am 2018;100(3):180–8.

12. Finney FT, Gossett TD, Hu HM, et al. New persistent opioid use following common forefoot procedures for the treatment of hallux valgus. J Bone Joint Surg Am 2019;101(8):722–9.

13. Rogero R, Fuchs D, Nicholson K, et al. Postoperative opioid consumption in Opioid-Naïve patients undergoing hallux valgus correction. Foot Ankle Int 2019; 40(11):1267–72.

14. Martin BC, Fan MY, Edlund MJ, et al. Long-term chronic opioid therapy discontinuation rates from the TROUP study. J Gen Intern Med 2011;26(12):1450–7.

15. Krischak GD, Augat P, Blakytny R, et al. The non-steroidal anti-inflammatory drug diclofenac reduces appearance of osteoblasts in bone defect healing in rats. Arch Orthop Trauma Surg 2007;127(6):453–8.

16. Wheatley BM, Nappo KE, Christensen DL, et al. Effect of NSAIDs on bone healing rates: a meta-analysis. J Am Acad Orthop Surg 2019;27(7):e330–6.

17. Pountos I, Georgouli T, Calori GM, et al. Do nonsteroidal anti-inflammatory drugs affect bone healing? A critical analysis. ScientificWorldJournal 2012;2012: 606404.

18. Lisowska B, Kosson D, Domaracka K. Positives and negatives of nonsteroidal anti-inflammatory drugs in bone healing: the effects of these drugs on bone repair. Drug Des Devel Ther 2018;12:1809–14.

19. Hassan MK, Karlock LG. The effect of post-operative NSAID administration on bone healing after elective foot and ankle surgery. Foot Ankle Surg, in press.

20. Mattila K, Kontinen VK, Kalso E, et al. Dexamethasone decreases oxycodone consumption following osteotomy of the first metatarsal bone: a randomized controlled trial in day surgery. Acta Anaesthesiol Scand 2010;54(3):268–76.

21. Henzi I, Walder B, Tramer MR. Dexamethasone for the prevention of postoperative nausea and vomiting: a quantitative systematic review. Anesth Analg 2000; 90(1):186–94.

22. Sauerland S, Nagelschmidt M, Mallmann P, et al. Risks and benefits of preoperative high dose methylprednisolone in surgical patients: a systematic review. Drug Saf 2000;23(5):449–61.

23. Sangeorzan BJ, Hansen ST Jr. Modified lapidus procedure for hallux valgus. Foot Ankle 1989;9(6):262–6.

24. Bednarz PA, Manoli A 2nd. Modified lapidus procedure for the treatment of hypermobile hallux valgus. Foot Ankle Int 2000;21(10):816–21.

25. Coughlin MJ, Mann RA, Saltzman CL. Surgery of the foot and ankle. 8th edition. Philadelphia: Mosby; 2007.

26. Pentikainen I, Piippo J, Ohtonen P, et al. Role of fixation and postoperative regimens in the long-term outcomes of distal chevron osteotomy: a randomized controlled two-by-two factorial trial of 100 patients. J Foot Ankle Surg 2015; 54(3):356–60.

27. Basile P, Cook EA, Cook JJ. Immediate weight bearing following modified lapidus arthrodesis. J Foot Ankle Surg 2010;49(5):459–64.

28. Kazzaz S, Singh D. Postoperative cast necessity after a lapidus arthrodesis. Foot Ankle Int 2009;30(8):746–51.

29. Ponzio DY, Pedowitz DI, Verma K, et al. Radiographic outcomes of postoperative taping following hallux valgus correction. Foot Ankle Int 2015;36(7):820–6.

30. Yucel I, Tenekecioglu Y, Ogut T, et al. Treatment of hallux valgus by modified McBride procedure: a 6-year follow-up. J Orthop Traumatol 2010;11(2):89–97.

31. Mittal D, Raja S, Geary NP. The modified McBride procedure: clinical, radiological, and pedobarographic evaluations. J Foot Ankle Surg 2006;45(4):235–9.

32. Stukenborg-Colsman C, Claaßen L, Ettinger S, et al. Distale Korrekturosteotomie zur Behandlung des Hallux valgus (Chevron-Osteotomie). Der Orthopäde 2017; 46(5):402–7.

33. Johnson JE, Clanton TO, Baxter DE, et al. Comparison of Chevron osteotomy and modified McBride bunionectomy for correction of mild to moderate hallux valgus deformity. Foot Ankle 1991;12(2):61–8.

34. Coetzee JC. Scarf osteotomy for hallux valgus repair: the dark side. Foot Ankle Int 2003;24(1):29–33.

35. Fraissler L, Konrads C, Hoberg M, et al. Treatment of hallux valgus deformity. EFORT Open Rev 2016;1(8):295–302.

36. Liszka H, Gadek A. Results of scarf osteotomy without implant fixation in the treatment of hallux valgus. Foot Ankle Int 2018;39(11):1320–7.

37. Nery C, Ressio C, de Azevedo Santa Cruz G, et al. Proximal opening-wedge osteotomy of the first metatarsal for moderate and severe hallux valgus using low profile plates. Foot Ankle Surg 2013;19(4):276–82.

38. Catanzariti AR, Mendicino RW, Lee MS, et al. The modified Lapidus arthrodesis: a retrospective analysis. J Foot Ankle Surg 1999;38(5):322–32.

39. Crowell A, Van JC, Meyr AJ. Early weightbearing after arthrodesis of the first metatarsal-medial cuneiform joint: a systematic review of the incidence of nonunion. J Foot Ankle Surg 2018;57(6):1204–6.

40. Ray JJ, Koay J, Dayton PD, et al. Multicenter early radiographic outcomes of triplanar tarsometatarsal arthrodesis with early weightbearing. Foot Ankle Int 2019; 40(8):955–60.

41. King CM, Richey J, Patel S, et al. Modified lapidus arthrodesis with crossed screw fixation: early weightbearing in 136 patients. J Foot Ankle Surg 2015;54(1):69–75.

42. Schuh R, Hofstaetter SG, Adams SB Jr, et al. Rehabilitation after hallux valgus surgery: importance of physical therapy to restore weight bearing of the first ray during the stance phase. Phys Ther 2009;89(9):934–45.

43. Jones S, Al Hussainy HA, Ali F, et al. Scarf osteotomy for hallux valgus. A prospective clinical and pedobarographic study. J Bone Joint Surg Br 2004;86(6): 830–6.

44. Bryant AR, Tinley P, Cole JH. Plantar pressure and radiographic changes to the forefoot after the Austin bunionectomy. J Am Podiatr Med Assoc 2005;95(4): 357–65.

45. Dhanendran M, Pollard JP, Hutton WC. Mechanics of the hallux valgus foot and the effect of Keller's operation. Acta Orthop Scand 1980;51(6):1007–12.

46. Dhukaram V, Hullin MG, Senthil Kumar C. The Mitchell and Scarf osteotomies for hallux valgus correction: a retrospective, comparative analysis using plantar pressures. J Foot Ankle Surg 2006;45(6):400–9.

47. Coetzee JC, Wickum D. The Lapidus procedure: a prospective cohort outcome study. Foot Ankle Int 2004;25(8):526–31.

48. MacMahon A, Karbassi J, Burket JC, et al. Return to sports and physical activities after the modified lapidus procedure for hallux valgus in young patients. Foot Ankle Int 2016;37(4):378–85.

49. McDonald E, Shakked R, Daniel J, et al. Driving after hallux valgus surgery. Foot Ankle Int 2017;38(9):982–6.

50. Holt G, Kay M, McGrory R, et al. Emergency brake response time after first metatarsal osteotomy. J Bone Joint Surg Am 2008;90(8):1660–4.

51. Dammerer D, Braito M, Biedermann R, et al. Effect of surgical shoes on brake response time after first metatarsal osteotomy–a prospective cohort study. J Orthop Surg Res 2016;11:14.

Management of Complications After Hallux Valgus Reconstruction

Manuel Monteagudo, MD[a,b,]*, Pilar Martínez-de-Albornoz, MD[a,b]

KEYWORDS

- Hallux valgus • Complications • Recurrence • Transfer metatarsalgia • Hallux varus
- Metatarsal osteotomy

KEY POINTS

- Complications following hallux valgus (HV) reconstruction will have an expected incidence of between 10% and 55% of cases.
- The more commonly reported complications include undercorrection/recurrence, overcorrection (hallux varus), transfer metatarsalgia, nonunion, malunion, avascular necrosis, arthritis, hardware removal, nerve injury, and ultimately patient dissatisfaction.
- Identification and hierarchization of the mechanical impairments involved in each particular case is critical to plan for the optimal management.
- The presence of arthritis will be an indication for fusion, whereas osteotomies will be the procedure of choice if the first metatarsophalangeal joint is healthy.
- Tendon transfers or tenodesis are useful as joint preserving procedures in iatrogenic hallux varus.

 Video content accompanies this article at http://www.foot.theclinics.com.

INTRODUCTION

Reconstructive hallux valgus (HV) surgery is one of the most common procedures in our foot and ankle practice. More than 100 surgical techniques have been described for hallux correction, some of which are no longer in use. Complications following HV reconstruction will have an expected incidence of between 10% and 55% of cases.[1] The more commonly reported complications include undercorrection, recurrence, overcorrection (hallux varus), transfer metatarsalgia, nonunion, malunion, avascular necrosis, arthritis, hardware removal, nerve injury, and ultimately patient dissatisfaction.[2] Sometimes these complications are asymptomatic,

[a] Orthopaedic Foot and Ankle Unit, Orthopaedic and Trauma Department, Hospital Universitario Quironsalud Madrid, Calle Diego de Velázquez 1, Madrid 28223, Spain; [b] Faculty of Medicine, UEM Madrid, Madrid, Spain
* Corresponding author.
E-mail address: mmontyr@yahoo.com

Foot Ankle Clin N Am 25 (2020) 151–167
https://doi.org/10.1016/j.fcl.2019.10.011
1083-7515/20/© 2019 Elsevier Inc. All rights reserved.

but frequently they render a first metatarsal that is painful and/or unable to function properly.

Management of suboptimal results following surgical treatment of HV deformity is challenging even to the experienced foot and ankle surgeon. A thorough understanding of the pathomechanics and biologics underlying the failed hallux is fundamental to plan proper treatment. If conservative measures fail to relieve pain, revision surgery may be indicated. In some cases, a successful outcome may be expected from revision of the first ray alone, but in some other cases surgery on the lesser rays or both combined may be necessary to achieve a mechanically sound forefoot.

Excluded in this work is the discussion of other general complications that may also need treatment: hematoma, complex regional pain syndrome, trauma, and thrombophlebitis. Arthritis, avascular necrosis, nonunion, and malunion will be explained in depth in Jorge Filippi and Jorge Briceno's article, "Complications after Metatarsal Osteotomies for Hallux Valgus: Malunion, Nonunion, Avascular Necrosis, and Metatarsophalangeal Osteoarthritis," in this issue. We will concentrate on addressing conservative and surgical management of failed hallux reconstruction, resulting in undercorrection/recurrence, overcorrection (hallux varus), transfer metatarsalgia, hardware removal, nerve injury, and patient dissatisfaction.

UNDERSTANDING COMPLICATIONS AND PLANNING MANAGEMENT

A recent systematic review of the literature reveals a pooled rate of postoperative patient dissatisfaction of 10.6% and residual first metatarsophalangeal (MP) pain of 1.5% after HV surgery.[3] Rates of revision surgery are higher for proximal procedures (closing base wedge osteotomy: 8.82%; Lapidus: 8.19%) than for distal techniques (Chevron: 5.56%).[4] However, it is almost impossible to get a precise picture of complications, as HV management has evolved from joint hemiresection (Keller-Brandes being no longer in use as a primary technique) to osteotomies and arthrodesis with those techniques being performed either minimally invasively or open and with or without implants. The authors describe correlations between the preoperative setting and the most common postoperative complications and suggest strategies for the management of these unfavorable results.

Conservative Management of Complications

Regardless the cause of a failed hallux, nonsurgical treatments should always be attempted, as they do not compromise future surgical revision. Treatment can include analgesics, offloading the painful first metatarsal or the lesser metatarsals by means of padding, orthoses, and/or adapted shoewear modification. However, there is no evidence to confirm the effectiveness of conservative measures for the treatment of most HV complications.[5] Functional orthoses may be helpful to control abnormal hindfoot pronation or supination that may alleviate pain around the failed hallux or iatrogenic metatarsalgia. A metatarsal raise just proximal to lesser metatarsal heads on the insole or orthoses may distribute force away from the head of an excessively long metatarsal after first metatarsal shortening. A wider toe box may relieve pain in patients with recurrence/under- and overcorrection. Rocker-bottom shoes seem to improve transition from the first to the third rocker and may alleviate pain around the hallux.[6] Rocker soles are particularly useful in the presence of an iatrogenic hallux limitus or rigidus or for postoperative stiffness of the first MP joint behaving mechanically as a hallux limitus/rigidus.

Surgical Management of Complications

If symptoms persist despite conservative measures, the revision surgical procedure should be chosen according to the same criteria than for the primary HV deformity. Several factors should be considered before setting up the correct indication for treatment:

1. Patient: surgery should not be considered if expectations are unrealistic. Arthrodesis may be a reasonable salvage option in older patients with poor bone stock regardless the state of the joint.
2. First MP joint: whatever the complication present, arthritis in the first MP joint should be an indication for fusion. Arthritis of plantar aspect of the first metatarsal head in contact with the sesamoids is sometimes only evident on a computed tomographic (CT) scan and may cause residual pain if an osteotomy is chosen as the salvage procedure (**Fig. 1**). First MP fusion has demonstrated good or excellent outcomes as a revision procedure in 72% of patients with a long follow-up.[7] Iliac crest grafting permits the restoration of the appropriate metatarsal length and the biology in cases of nonunion. Lapidus arthrodesis is the procedure of choice if clinical hypermobility of the first tarsometatarsal joint or flatfoot deformity are present (**Fig. 2**).[8]

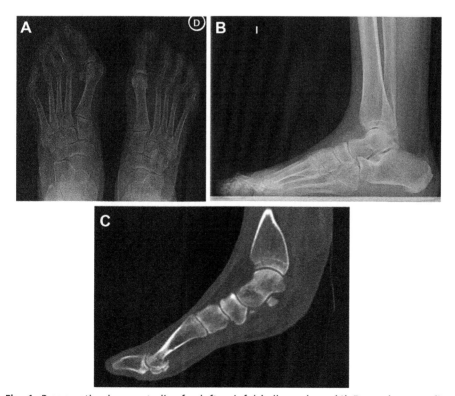

Fig. 1. Preoperative image studies for left painful hallux valgus. (*A*) Dorsoplantar radiograph of weight-bearing feet showing hallux valgus with no apparent signs of arthritis. (*B*) Lateral radiograph of the same patient with no signs of arthritis. (*C*) Sagittal CT image demonstrate extensive arthritis in the plantar aspect of the first metatarsal head and the sesamoids.

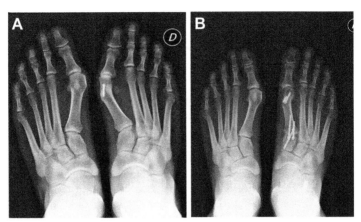

Fig. 2. Failed HV surgery. (*A*) Undercorrection following distal first metatarsal osteotomy in a patient with hypermobility of the first tarsometatarsal joint. (*B*) Revision surgery with Lapidus arthrodesis.

If the joint is "healthy," a joint-preserving osteotomy should be planned to place the metatarsal head over the sesamoids and to adjust the relative length of the first metatarsal with respect to the second (ideally an index plus minus formula). The choice of a particular osteotomy depends on the type and magnitude of correction needed but also on the particular experience of the surgeon. A common mistake is trying to repair our own failed HV case (and our ego) by performing a less powerful revision osteotomy than needed in the new setting.

3. Surgeon: the inappropriate choice of a procedure at index surgery is a common cause of failure. Keller-Brandes joint hemiresection has historically shown poor results and has been associated with the highest rate of postoperative transfer metatarsalgia and patient dissatisfaction.[3,9] Wide experience in primary HV surgery is advised before dealing with complex cases of failed HV surgery.

4. Joint congruity and soft tissue balancing: when the joint is flexible and have no arthritic signs, joint mobility may be improved by restoring its congruity. Wedged osteotomies (distal first metatarsal or proximal phalanx) may improve the distal metatarsal articular angle and favor better mechanics at the MP1 joint. Soft tissue balancing is especially important when dealing with flexible, nonarthritic, overcorrection resulting in painful hallux varus.

Although patient considerations and the state of the first MP are important factors to decide which would be the optimal treatment of the failed hallux, it is important to consider each of the particular situations leading to failure to contemplate some particular variants of treatment strategies.

Most complications/errors after HV surgery are a consequence of the following:

- Operating the hallux that should not be operated (ie, cosmetic HV surgery).
- Operating in the wrong anatomic location (ie, flatfoot deformity with secondary HV).
- Producing an undesirable mechanical effect (ie, shortening and/or elevation of the first metatarsal resulting in transfer metatarsalgia).
- Producing a mechanical effect in an undesirable magnitude (ie, undercorrection/overcorrection).

The first 2 considerations correspond to errors of indication. The last 2 considerations correspond to errors of planning and/or execution (surgical technique).

OPERATING ON THE HALLUX THAT SHOULD NOT BE OPERATED ON

In 2005, AOFAS (American Orthopedic Foot Ankle Society) Board of Directors approved a statement over cosmetic surgery of the foot and ankle.[10] *"There exists no literature to support operating on a bunion deformity in an asymptomatic forefoot. The existing medical literature ..."* However, we still have to spend time every week explaining the occasional patient not to have surgery in her/his asymptomatic "not-so-beautiful" HV.

OPERATING IN THE WRONG ANATOMIC LOCATION

Flat foot deformity has been described as a risk factor for failure in HV surgery. Although some investigators state that the presence of flatfeet does not reduce the success rate of operations for HV,[11] progression of HV is more rapid in patients with flatfeet.[12] When they have failed to address a symptomatic flatfoot deformity with HV, a high rate of recurrence is observed. Malunion in valgus of different types of peritalar osteotomies and fusions should also be addressed before surgery of an HV.

PRODUCING AN UNDESIRABLE MECHANICAL EFFECT

The term *transfer metatarsalgia* refers to the onset of pain at a different ray than that which is mechanically impaired. HV surgery may impair first ray function and produce signs and symptoms at any other region around the lesser MP joints.

Between 11% and 20% of patients may develop transfer metatarsalgia following Mitchell's osteotomy.[13] Wilson and Mitchell osteotomies are prone to shortening the first metatarsal.[14] But it seems that the rate of postoperative transfer metatarsalgia is highest in patients who underwent joint hemiresection.[3]

Surgical planning of transfer metatarsalgia post-HV surgery would start by addressing the state of the first metatarsal. In many cases, revision surgery of the first ray will restore function and resolve lesser metatarsals overload.[9] Reconstruction of the first ray may restore forefoot biomechanics provided a harmonic metatarsal parabola is recreated, but lesser metatarsal surgery is sometimes necessary. Recurrence of the deformity and shortening of the first metatarsal are the most common causes of transfer metatarsalgia.[9] First ray insufficiency may cause overload of the central rays during the third rocker (**Fig. 3**). Depending on how the lesser metatarsals cope with this overload, several scenarios may develop. A second metatarsal stress fracture may be the result of shortening and elevation of the first metatarsal head (ie, troughing in scarf osteotomy). Second space syndrome, with divergent second and third toes due to adduction at the second MP joint, can be due to an excessively long second metatarsal with respect to an iatrogenically shortened first metatarsal. Although some investigators[13–15] advocate lengthening step-cut osteotomies, the authors prefer shortening of the lesser rays or bone block arthrodesis if the joint is arthritic. Lengthening of an iatrogenically shortened first metatarsal may favor the development of a functional hallux limitus or ultimately hallux rigidus, metatarsal head necrosis, arthritis, or postoperative first metatarsal stress fracture (**Fig. 4**).

Elevation will cause the first MP joint to plantarflex to compensate for metatarsal elevation, and the hallucal interphalangeal joint will dorsiflex to help with push off at

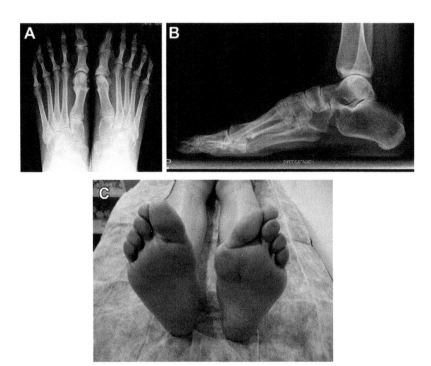

Fig. 3. Common complications after HV surgery. (*A*) Dorsoplantar radiograph shows shortening and metatarsal arthritis following mini-invasive surgery of both first metatarsals. (*B*) Lateral radiograph reveals distal elevation of the metatarsal head. (*C*) Both feet present with central keratosis in the metatarsal region as a result of first ray mechanical insufficiency due to shortening and elevation.

the third rocker. Traction sesamoiditis may arise. Iatrogenic elevation of the first metatarsal after distal metaphyseal osteotomies may be managed by performing a plantar-flexion opening wedge osteotomy (base dorsal, apex plantar) and inserting a corticocancellous bone graft.[16] Elevation is frequently associated with shortening. This combination is commonly seen after procedures performed in the proximal region

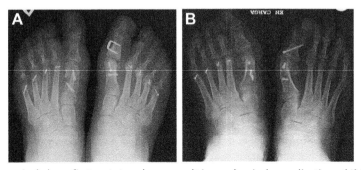

Fig. 4. Excessively long first metatarsal may result in mechanical complications. (*A*) Note the different metatarsal parabola between both feet, with arthritis in the long first metatarsal after forefoot reconstruction in the right foot. (*B*) Postoperative stress fracture of the first metatarsal due to excessive length with respect to the second.

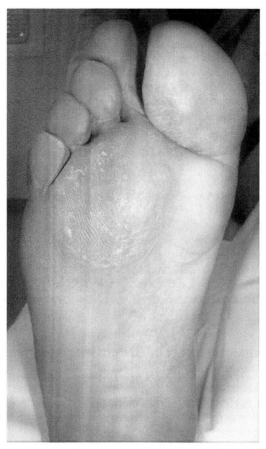

Fig. 5. Midfoot pronation after first metatarsal elevation will result in lesser metatarsal overload with a typical keratosis.

of the first metatarsal (basal wedge osteotomy, Lapidus arthrodesis). Midfoot pronation together with an iatrogenic hallux limitus may cause a third rocker overload at the fourth and fifth metatarsals (**Fig. 5**).

An excessive iatrogenic first metatarsal plantarflexion is rare.[16] In the presence of an excessively plantarflexed first metatarsal, midfoot supination with second rocker overload at the fifth metatarsal may be expected. Second rocker overload under the first metatarsal head combined with compression sesamoiditis will possibly be symptomatic. In this setting, a dorsiflexion osteotomy of the first metatarsal should be considered.

If we focus on the possible surgical procedures for the lesser metatarsals, identification of the type of transfer metatarsalgia is crucial for the choice of the correct procedure:

1. *Iatrogenic second rocker metatarsalgia* would be the result of an abnormal loading in the sagittal plane (during the second rocker of gait) and would respond to dorsiflexion/elevating osteotomies of the lesser metatarsal. Traditionally, proximal osteotomies (ie, Goldbarb or Barouk-Rippstein-Toullec) produced a dorsiflexion wedge in the proximal metaphysis of an excessively plantarflexed lesser metatarsal to relieve localized metatarsalgia. However, there

is no way to quantify the exact amount of dorsiflexion together with each metatarsal individual motion in the sagittal plane, thus it is frequent to induce a second rocker transfer metatarsalgia. Alternatively, a distal tilt-up osteotomy with a dorsal extraarticular wedge may restore the height of the second metatarsal head and allow for chondral reorientation (as for Freiberg disease) with less variability in the magnitude of the sagittal correction.[9]

2. *Iatrogenic third rocker metatarsalgia* may be managed by the use of distal metatarsal osteotomies, such as the Weil and the triple Weil osteotomies, designed to restore the ideal metatarsal parabola and redistribute weight-bearing forces around the forefoot.

Keller bunionectomy was frequently associated with metatarsal shortening, first ray dysfunction, transfer metatarsalgia, and stress fractures of lesser metatarsals.[17] Revision surgery for a failed Keller usually includes first MP joint fusion and lesser metatarsal osteotomies or head resection.[18,19] If there is no pain at the failed first MP joint and there is a short first metatarsal (index minus), quantified triple Weil osteotomies of the lesser rays may be enough to deal with transfer metatarsalgia.

Panmetatarsal head resections play an important role in the management of the rheumatoid patient with a failed HV surgery.[20] If the failed hallux shows signs of arthritis and there are severe fixed deformities involving all MP joints, the combination of a first MP joint fusion and panmetatarsal head resection could restore a pain-free forefoot (**Fig. 6**).

PRODUCING A MECHANICAL EFFECT IN AN UNDESIRABLE MAGNITUDE
Undercorrection/Recurrence

Reduction of the first metatarsal over the sesamoids is capital to achieve a correct mechanical alignment in HV surgery. Undercorrection and recurrence are different entities. When considering *recurrence* it is assumed the first metatarsal was in place for a time with disappearance of HV and then reduction was lost overtime. Undercorrection means the first metatarsal was never reduced and HV was to a degree always present from surgery (**Fig. 7**).

Recurrence is one of the most common complications after HV surgery with an estimated rate of up to 16% and the cause is multifactorial.[21] Several investigators[21,22] have studied the potential causes for recurrence and they may be divided into the following:

1. *Local anatomic* (skeletal immaturity, incongruent joint [high distal metatarsal articular angle], lateral slope of the articular surface, metatarsal head dysplasia, metatarsus adductus, hindfoot deformities) (**Fig. 8**). Adolescent HV surgery presents with lower rates of recurrence (8%) and other complications than the historically reported figures.[23] Hypermobility of the first tarsometatarsal joint remains a controversial factor, but a higher recurrence rate may be expected in patients with this condition.[24]

2. *Social* (noncompliant postop management, inadequate shoewear). Continued wear of high-heel and narrow toe box following correction may predispose to recurrence.[21]

3. *Systemic* (neuromuscular condition, pathologic hyperlaxity [Ehlers-Danlos, Marfan), rheumatoid arthritis, seronegative arthropathies, gout). Inflammatory arthritis and neuromuscular conditions may cause loss of correction.[22]

4. *Surgical* (wrong surgical planning and technique, nonunion, infection). Wrong preoperative planning and/or inadequate surgical technique may favor recurrence.

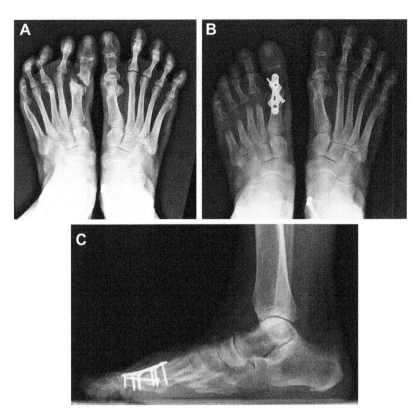

Fig. 6. Complications after forefoot reconstruction. (*A*) The left first MP joint shows advanced arthritis. Deformities and articular damage were also present in the lesser MP joints. (*B*) Dorsoplantar radiograph showing panmetatarsal head resection with first MP fusion performed as a salvage procedure. (*C*) Lateral radiograph of the same patient.

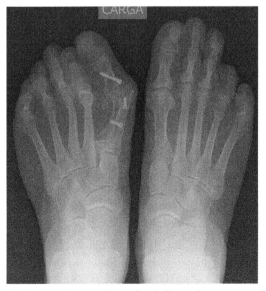

Fig. 7. Radiograph showing undercorrection after hallux valgus surgery that resulted in progressive dislocations of the lesser MP joints.

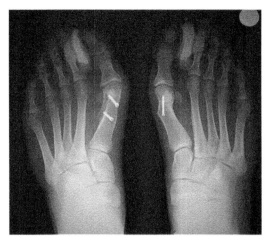

Fig. 8. Abnormal shape of the lateral slope of the articular first MP surface (left foot) may predispose to recurrence.

Inadequate lateral soft tissue release (Videos 1 and 2) (possibly the most common cause of undercorrection), incongruent joint, isolated bunionectomy, incomplete reduction of first metatarsal over the sesamoids, inability to recreate the correct metatarsal parabola (ie, index plus), are all associated with a higher risk of HV recurrence.[22]

The literature on the treatment of recurrent HV is sparse.[22] Lagaay and colleagues[4] could not find a significant difference in revision rates over the various methods/techniques of primary HV correction. Most papers analyzing failures of HV surgery do not address the severity of the deformity before the index procedure or why a particular technique was indicated.[3,21]

Many patients with undercorrection have little or no pain, so revision surgery is not recommended. If symptomatic, and in the absence of other disturbing factors (arthritis, poor bone stock), revision surgery would include removal of metalwork, a correct lateral release, and a new osteotomy that allows the correct positioning of the metatarsal head over the sesamoids (**Fig. 9**). Recurrence associated with first MP arthritis is best managed with first MP fusion. Arthritis of the first tarsometatarsal joint is an indication for Lapidus procedure and has proved to be a reliable and effective operation after failed HV surgery in appropriately selected cases.[24,25] Index plus (with iatrogenic long first metatarsal) may be managed with a shortening/repositioning first metatarsal osteotomy. Additional procedures around the hallux (Akin osteotomy, lesser metatarsal osteotomies in the presence of a too short first metatarsal) may be needed in some cases and should be planned beforehand on the preoperative weight-bearing radiographs. Follow-up of at least a year is necessary to rule out recurrence in both primary and revision surgery.

Overcorrection—Hallux Varus

McBride[26] first reported an incidence of 5% of iatrogenic hallux varus following his technique combining bunionectomy, medial capsulorrhaphy, and fibular sesamoid excision. But overcorrection after HV surgery resulting in hallux varus has been reported to range from 2% to 17%.[27] The causes of hallux varus include systemic inflammatory disorders, Charcot-Marie-Tooth disease, avascular necrosis of the first

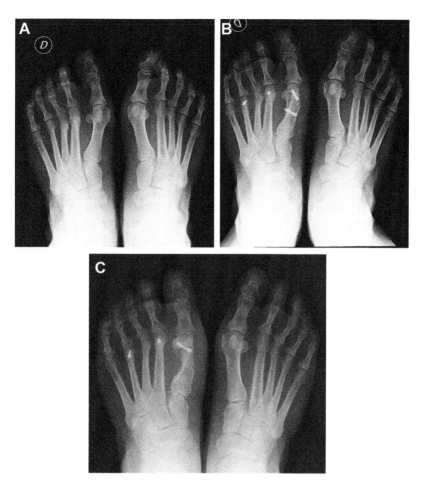

Fig. 9. Mixed (second and third rocker) metatarsalgia may be explained by suboptimal results after metatarsal mini-invasive osteotomies without hallux correction. (*A*) Dorsoplantar radiograph reveals abnormal metatarsal parabola and hallux valgus. (*B*) Revision surgery with a harmonic metatarsal parabola but undercorrected hallux. (*C*) New revision surgery was needed for hallux correction.

metatarsal head, trauma, and polio. However, hallux varus is most commonly the result of overcorrection in HV surgery and is highest in patients who underwent a proximal osteotomy.[28]

Many patients with hallux varus are asymptomatic and do not need treatment, particularly in the absence of arthritis of the first MP joint and a mild deformity (<10°).[29] But some patients present with transfer metatarsalgia or pain around the hallux (**Fig. 10**). Cosmetic deformity and difficulty fitting into conventional footwear are other common complaints.

Pathogenesis of iatrogenic hallux varus is complex, and many factors may contribute to the final deformity: excessive lateral release, excessive tightening of the medial structures, aggressive postoperative bandaging holding the toe in a varus position, fibular sesamoidectomy, excessive resection of the medial eminence, and excessive lateral displacement of an osteotomy (**Fig. 11**).[30]

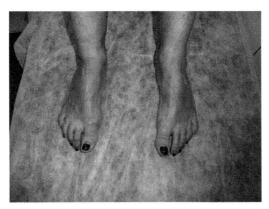

Fig. 10. Left hallux varus produced secondary supination of the forefoot and midfoot with lateral metatarsal overload.

Early recognition of iatrogenic hallux varus may benefit from dressing and tapings, but those measures are only effective when they are applied within the first 2 to 3 weeks from surgery and in less than a quarter of cases.[31]

Surgical treatment of iatrogenic hallux varus should seek a functional, painless, and shoeable foot while maintaining or restoring joint mobility whenever possible. In all cases, medial capsular release is necessary for rest of the surgical techniques to work. Decision-making over which technique to choose depends on the state of the following:

1. Joint: if there is arthritis and/or a rigid contracture of the joint then arthrodesis should be the procedure of choice.

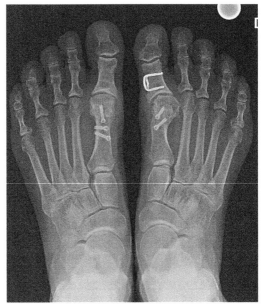

Fig. 11. Bilateral hallux varus after excessive lateral displacement of first metatarsal osteotomies.

2. First metatarsal: excessive bone resection at the medial eminence after an aggressive bunionectomy may be overcome by bone grafting.[32] Distal Chevron metatarsal osteotomies to reverse overcorrection have been advocated with apparent good results.[1,33] Kannegieter and Kilmartin[34] combined a stepwise approach for patients with a combination of scarf and Akin osteotomies, with all 5 patients in their series being satisfied after the procedure.

3. Soft tissue: in nonarthritic joints, there is evidence to suggest that lateral capsule imbrication, conjoined adductor tendon repair and tightening, and medial capsule and abductor tendon release are unsuccessful in correcting hallux varusdeformity.[35,36] The most popular soft tissue repair for hallux varus—extensor hallucis longus (with fusion of the interphalangeal joint)—was reviewed by Plovanich and colleagues[37] including 8 studies with an overall complication rate of 16.6% and recurrence of HV in 4.4% of cases.

Tendon transfers around the hallux varus look for the dynamic correction of the deformity:

- Hawkins[35] proposed the release of the abductor tendon from the base of the proximal phalanx, its routing beneath the intermetatarsal ligament, and fixation to the lateral side of the base of the phalanx. Potential supination of the toe and difficulty with harvesting the tendon are concerns over this technique.
- Valtin[38] described the transferring of the first dorsal interosseous tendon to the base of the proximal phalanx through a bone tunnel. Drawbacks of the technique include the potential effects on the second toe and the difficulty in the reinsertion of such a small tendon.
- Johnson and Spiegl[39] proposed a transfer of the entire extensor hallucis longus tendon, beneath the first intermetatarsal ligament, to the plantar-lateral area of the proximal phalanx. The reduced residual extension of the hallux and the loss of interphalangeal motion made interphalangeal fusion a necessity to avoid the development of a mallet toe. To avoid fusion of the interphalangeal joint, the same investigators modified the original technique by using a split-lateral-half of the extensor hallucis longus for the transfer and leaving the medial half untouched. However, tension applied to the lateral portion of the tendon is also transferred to the remaining medial half, thus altering its function.

Tenodesis around the hallux varus look for the static correction of the deformity:

- To avoid altering the mechanics of the remaining extensor hallucis tendon and provide a more reliable correction, Lau and Myerson[40] recommended detaching the lateral half of the extensor hallucis longus tendon proximally and passing it from distal to proximal under the intermetatarsal ligament of the first web space and fixed medially through an osseous tunnel in the neck of the first metatarsal with the hallux in the corrected position.
- Juliano and colleagues[36] described an extensor hallucis brevis tenodesis in which the tendon is transected at the musculotendinous junction and passed plantar to the intermetatarsal ligament and reattached through a bone tunnel from lateral to medial on the first metatarsal. A potential advantage of this technique is the preservation of the extension function of the distal phalanx. The investigators reported an excellent correction in 6 cases of hallux varus. Myerson and Komenda[41] also found the same excellent results in 6 patients using this technique.
- Leemrijse and colleagues[42] developed an anatomic tenodesis by using one-third of the abductor hallucis tendon detached proximally and released from the tibial

sesamoid. The tendon is passed through 2 osseous tunnels, from medial to lateral in the proximal phalanx and then from lateral to medial through the first metatarsal. Good maintenance of the correction was obtained in 7 patients who underwent this type of tenodesis.

The lateral ligamentous structures may also be reconstructed as an alternative to tendon transfer or tenodesis with Ligapro suture[43] or soft tissue anchors.[44] Some investigators have reported on the use of a button and suture technique for the correction of hallux varus.[45,46] Potential complications include fractures of the phalanx or metatarsal and loss of correction if the suture device breaks before sufficient lateral scarring has taken place.

OTHER (LESS COMMON) COMPLICATIONS
Nerve Injury

Loss of sensation and formation of a neuroma are potential complications of HVsurgery.[47] Sensory loss was reported by Campbell in 45% of operations.[48] Meier and Kenzora[49] reported an incidence of painful scars of 5% in their series. In a recent systematic literature review, the rate of intraoperative nerve injury was comparable across all surgery types averaging 3%.[3,47] The surgical release of the dorsomedial cutaneous nerve from fibrotic surrounding tissue may relieve pain in some patients (Video 3).[50]

Hardware Removal

Although the introduction (during the 1990s) of internal fixation for the treatment of HV led to the reduction of overall complication rates (especially arthritis and transfer metatarsalgia associated to joint hemiresection procedures), hardware-related pain is a potential complication. Apparently, the more the hardware used (first tarsometatarsal arthrodesis and first MP arthrodesis), the higher the rate of secondary surgery for removal.[3]

Patient Dissatisfaction

In a systematic review of the literature analyzing unfavorable outcomes following HVsurgery,[3] dissatisfaction after HV surgery is apparently highest in patients who underwent joint hemiresection or a simple bunionectomy. In the same study, patients with lower preoperative intermetatarsal angles were more dissatisfied than patients with higher angles. Overall dissatisfaction rate was 10.6%, something not to be ignored by surgeons.

Infectious/Skin/Vascular

Infection seems to be more common after first tarsometatarsal fusion (Lapidus) and very uncommon after a metatarsal shaft osteotomy.[3] Septic arthritis following HV surgery may be managed by staged arthrodesis—first stage for debridement with antibiotic cement spacer followed by a second stage for spacer removal and tricortical iliac crest grafting.[51,52] Myerson and colleagues[51] reported control of the infection in 5 patients although nonunion of the graft proximally was registered in 2 patients.

Dayton and colleagues[53] studied the safety of suture techniques to reduce the intermetatarsal angle in HV surgery to find a pooled rate of complications of 19.8%, including fractures (10.7%), hardware failure (5.6%), and hallux varus (3.6%). The use of certain barbed sutures for knotless wound closure has been associated with delayed wound healing and superficial dermal abscess formation.[54]

SUMMARY

Complications following HV reconstruction will have an expected incidence of between 10% and 55% of cases. The more commonly reported complications include undercorrection/recurrence, overcorrection (hallux varus), transfer metatarsalgia, nonunion, malunion, avascular necrosis, arthritis, hardware removal, nerve injury, and ultimately patient dissatisfaction. The presence of arthritis will be an indication for fusion, whereas osteotomies will be the procedure of choice if the first MP joint is healthy. Tendon transfers or tenodesis are useful as joint-preserving procedures in iatrogenic hallux varus. Revision surgery may be confined to the first ray or may need surgery in the lesser rays or even away from the forefoot. Patients' expectations should be realistic otherwise surgery should not be indicated. A common mistake is trying to repair a failed HV by performing a less powerful revision osteotomy than needed in the new setting. A big problem needs a big hammer. Wide experience in primary HV surgery is advised before dealing with complex cases of failed HV surgery.

DISCLOSURE

The authors have nothing to disclose.

SUPPLEMENTARY DATA

Supplementary data related to this article can be found online at https://doi.org/10.1016/j.fcl.2019.10.011.

REFERENCES

1. Lee KT, Park YU, Jegal H, et al. Deceptions in hallux valgus: what to look for to limit failures. Foot Ankle Clin 2014;19:361–70.
2. Baravarian B, Ben-Ad R. Revision hallux valgus: causes and correction options. Clin Podiatr Med Surg 2014;31(2):291–8.
3. Barg A, Harmer JR, Presson AP, et al. Unfavorable outcomes following surgical treatment of hallux valgus deformity: a systematic literature review. J Bone Joint Surg Am 2018;100:1563–73.
4. Lagaay PM, Hamilton GA, Ford LA, et al. Rates of revision surgery using Chevron-Austin osteotomy, Lapidus arthrodesis, and closing base wedge osteotomy for correction of hallux valgus deformity. J Foot Ankle Surg 2008;47(4):267–72.
5. Sammarco GJ, Idusuyi OB. Complications after surgery of the hallux. Clin Orthop Relat Res 2001;391:59–71.
6. Choi JY, Babu H, Joseph FN, et al. Effects of wearing shoes on the feet: Radiographic comparison of middle-aged partially shod Maasai women's feet and regularly shod Maasai and Korean women's feet. Foot Ankle Surg 2018;24(4):330–5.
7. Grimes JS, Coughlin MJ. First metatarsophalangeal joint arthrodesis as a treatment for failed hallux valgus surgery. Foot Ankle Int 2006;27(11):887–93.
8. Ellington JK, Myerson MS, Coetzee JC, et al. The use of the Lapidus procedure for recurrent hallux valgus. Foot Ankle Int 2011;32(7):674–80.
9. Maceira E, Monteagudo M. Transfer metatarsalgia post hallux valgus surgery. Foot Ankle Clin 2014;19(2):285–307.
10. AOFAS Board of Directors. Position statement cosmetic foot and ankle surgery 2015. Available at: https://www.aofas.org/docs/default-source/research-and-policy/position_statement_on_cosmetic_foot_and_ankle_surgery.pdf?sfvrsn=c416380b_2.

11. Ginés-Cespedosa A, Pérez-Prieto D, Muñetón D, et al. Influence of hindfootmala-lignment on hallux valgus operative outcomes. Foot Ankle Int 2016;37(8):842–7.
12. Scranton PE Jr, Pedegana LR, Whitesel JP. Gait analysis. Alterations in support phase forces using supportive devices. Am J Sports Med 1982;10(1):6–11.
13. Goldberg A, Singh D. Treatment of shortening following hallux valgus surgery. Foot Ankle Clin 2014;19(2):309–16.
14. Rose B, Bowman N, Edwards H, et al. Lengthening scarf osteotomy for recurrent hallux valgus. Foot Ankle Surg 2014;20(1):20–5.
15. Chowdhary A, Drittenbass L, Stern R, et al. Technique tip: Simultaneous first metatarsal lengthening and metatarsophalangeal joint fusion for failed hallux valgus surgery with transfer metatarsalgia. Foot Ankle Surg 2017;23(1):e8–11.
16. Caminear DS, Addis-Thomas E, Brynizcka AW, et al. Revision hallux valgus surgery. In: Saxena A, editor. Special procedures in foot and ankle surgery. London: Springer-Verlag; 2013. p. 17–35.
17. Friend G. Sequential metatarsal stress fractures after Keller arthroplasty with implant. J Foot Surg 1981;20:227–31.
18. Machacek F Jr, Easley ME, Gruber F, et al. Salvage of the failed Keller resection arthroplasty. J Bone Joint Surg Am 2004;86(6):1131–8.
19. Vienne P, Sukthankar A, Favre P, et al. Metatarsophalangeal joint arthrodesis after failed Keller-Brandes procedure. Foot Ankle Int 2006;27(11):894–901.
20. Molloy AP, Myerson MS. Surgery of the lesser toes in rheumatoid arthritis: meta-tarsal head resection. Foot Ankle Clin 2007;12:417–33.
21. Raikin SM, Miller AG, Daniel J. Recurrence of hallux valgus: a review. Foot Ankle Clin 2014;19(2):259–74.
22. Duan X, Kadakia AR. Salvage of recurrence after failed surgical treatment of hallux valgus. Arch Orthop Trauma Surg 2012;132(4):477–85.
23. Harb Z, Kokkinakis M, Ismail H, et al. Adolescent hallux valgus: a systematic re-view of outcomes following surgery. J Child Orthop 2015;9:105–12.
24. Coetzee JC, Resig SG, Kuskowski M, et al. The Lapidus procedure as salvage after failed surgical treatment of hallux valgus. Surgical technique. J Bone Joint Surg Am 2004;86-A(Suppl 1):30–6.
25. Espinosa N, Wirth SH. Tarsometatarsal arthrodesis for management of unstable first ray and failed bunion surgery. Foot Ankle Clin 2011;16(1):21–34.
26. McBride ED. The McBride bunion hallux valgus operation. J Bone Joint Surg Am 1967;49(8):1675–83.
27. Crawford MD, Patel J, Giza E. Iatrogenic hallux varus treatment algorithm. Foot Ankle Clin 2014;19(3):371–84.
28. Edelman RD. Iatrogenically induced hallux varus. Clin Podiatr Med Surg 1991; 8(2):367–82.
29. Trnka HJ, Zetti R, Hungerford M, et al. Acquired hallux varus and clinical tolera-bility. Foot Ankle Int 1997;18:593–7.
30. Davies MB, Blundell CM. The treatment of iatrogenic hallux varus. Foot Ankle Clin 2014;19(2):275–84.
31. Skalley TC, Myerson MS. The operative treatment of acquired hallux varus. Clin Orthop Relat Res 1994;(306):183–91.
32. Rochwerger A, Curvale G, Groulier P. Application of bone graft to the medial side of the first metatarsal head in the treatment of hallux varus. J Bone Joint Surg Am 1999;81(12):1730–5.
33. Choi KJ, Lee HS, Yoon YS, et al. Distal metatarsal osteotomy for hallux varus following surgery for hallux valgus. J Bone Joint Surg Br 2011;93(8):1079–83.

34. Kannegieter E, Kilmartin TE. The combined reverse scarf and opening wedge osteotomy of the proximal phalanx for the treatment of iatrogenic hallux varus. Foot (Edinb) 2011;21(2):88–91.
35. Hawkins FB. Acquired hallux varus: cause, prevention and correction. Clin Orthop Relat Res 1971;76:169–76.
36. Juliano PJ, Myerson MS, Cunningham BW. Biomechanical assessment of a new tenodesis for correction of hallux varus. Foot Ankle Int 1996;17(1):17–20.
37. Plovanich EJ, Donnenwerth MP, Abicht BP, et al. Failure after soft-tissue release with tendon transfer for flexible iatrogenic hallux varus: a systematic review. J Foot Ankle Surg 2012;51(2):195–7.
38. Valtin B. First dorsal interosseous muscle transfer in iatrogenic hallux varus surgery. Med Chir Pied 1991;7:9–16.
39. Johnson KA, Spiegl PV. Extensor hallucislongus transfer for hallux varus deformity. J Bone Joint Surg Am 1984;66(5):681–6.
40. Lau JT, Myerson MS. Modified split extensor hallucislongus tendon transfer for correction of hallux varus. Foot Ankle Int 2002;23(12):1138–40.
41. Myerson MS, Komenda GA. Results of hallux varus correction using an extensor hallucisbrevistenodesis. Foot Ankle Int 1996;17(1):21–7.
42. Leemrijse T, Hoang B, Maldague P, et al. A new surgical procedure for iatrogenic hallux varus: reverse transfer of the abductor hallucis tendon: a report of 7 cases. Acta Orthop Belg 2008;74(2):227–34.
43. Tourne Y, Saragaglia D, Picard F, et al. Iatrogenic hallux varus surgical procedure: a study of 14 cases. Foot Ankle Int 1995;16(8):457–63.
44. Labovitz JM, Kaczander BI. Traumatic hallux varus repair utilizing a soft-tissue anchor: a case report. J Foot Ankle Surg 2000;39(2):120–3.
45. Pappas AJ, Anderson RB. Management of acquired hallux varus with an Endobutton. Tech Foot Ankle Surg 2008;7(2):134–8.
46. Gerbert J, Traynor C, Blue K, et al. Use of the Mini TightRope® for correction of hallux varus deformity. J Foot Ankle Surg 2011;50(2):245–51.
47. Solan MC, Lemon M, Bendall SP. The surgical anatomy of the dorsomedial cutaneous nerve of the hallux. J Bone Joint Surg Br 2001;83:250–2.
48. Campbell DA. Sensory nerve damage during surgery on the hallux. J R Coll Surg Edinb 1992;37:422–4.
49. Meier PJ, Kenzora JE. The risks and benefits of distal first metatarsal osteotomies. Foot Ankle 1985;6(1):7–17.
50. Kenzora JE. Sensory nerve neuromas: leading to failed foot surgery. Foot Ankle 1986;7:110–7.
51. Myerson MS, Miller SD, Henderson MR, et al. Staged arthrodesis for salvage of the septic hallux metatarsophalangeal joint. Clin Orthop Relat Res 1994;307: 174–81.
52. Núñez-Samper M, Viladot R, Ponce SJ, et al. Serious sequellae of the hallux valgus surgery: More options for its surgical treatment. Rev Esp Cir Ortop Traumatol 2016;60(4):234–42.
53. Dayton P, Sedberry S, Feilmeier M. Complications of metatarsal suture techniques for bunion correction: a systematic review of the literature. J Foot Ankle Surg 2015;54(2):230–2.
54. Chowdhry M, Singh S. Severe scar problems following use of a locking barbed skin closure system in the foot. Foot Ankle Surg 2013;19(2):131–4.

Complications after Metatarsal Osteotomies for Hallux Valgus

Malunion, Nonunion, Avascular Necrosis, and Metatarsophalangeal Osteoarthritis

Jorge Filippi, MD, MBA[a],*, Jorge Briceno, MD[b]

KEYWORDS

- Hallux valgus complications • Metatarsal malunion • Metatarsal nonunion
- Metatarsal avascular necrosis • Hallux rigidus

KEY POINTS

- Metatarsal head avascular necrosis (AVN) can be effectively prevented avoiding extensive plantar bone stripping of the metatarsal neck. Also when a distal chevron osteotomy is performed, the plantar cut should finish well proximal to the capsular attachment in order to keep the plantar vascular supply of the metatarsal head.
- Nonunion is a very infrequent complication after metatarsal osteotomies. Intrinsic stability and location of the osteotomy, type of fixation, and comorbidities, including vitamin D deficiency, can influence the occurrence of this unusual situation.
- Malunion after hallux valgus surgery includes shortening, elevation, plantarflexion, varus/valgus, and rotational deformities. They can lead to pain, stiffness, deformity recurrence, and transfer metatarsalgia.
- First metatarsophalangeal (MTP) arthritis can be developed after metatarsal malunion or AVN. Treatment options include cheilectomy, osteotomies to correct malunions, and MTP arthrodesis.

INTRODUCTION

Hallux valgus (HV) is a common foot disorder. Its prevalence has been estimated between 23% and 35%.[1] Long-term studies with a follow-up time of 10 and 14 years have shown rates of radiological recurrence of around 30%.[2,3] Barg and colleagues,[4]

---

[a] Foot and Ankle Division, Department of Orthopedic Surgery, Clinica Las Condes, Estoril 450, Las Condes, Santiago 7591047, Chile; [b] Foot and Ankle Service, Department of Orthopedic Surgery, Pontificia Universidad Catolica de Chile, Diagonal Paraguay 362, Piso 3, Santiago 8330077, Chile
* Corresponding author.
E-mail address: jlfilippi@gmail.com

Foot Ankle Clin N Am 25 (2020) 169–182
https://doi.org/10.1016/j.fcl.2019.10.008
1083-7515/20/© 2019 Elsevier Inc. All rights reserved.

in a systematic review including a total of 229 studies, found a rate of postoperative patient dissatisfaction of 10.6%. Although most of the series show rates of clinical success of around 90%, many of them do not focus specifically on unfavorable outcomes.

The list of reported complications includes recurrence of hallux valgus deformity, persistent pain, transfer metatarsalgia, avascular necrosis (AVN), hallux varus, delayed union, nonunion, malunion of metatarsal osteotomies, wound healing problems, nerve injuries, infection, and painful stiffness.[2–7] Many of these complications can be prevented with adequate surgical planning, taking in consideration patient-related conditions such as age, bone quality, vitamin D status, and also technical considerations of the procedure, surgeon's experience, rehabilitation protocol, and giving realistic preoperative counseling of the results and recovery time to the patient.[8]

AVN, nonunion, malunion, and metatarsophalangeal (MTP) osteoarthritis following hallux valgus surgery, as well as pathophysiology, diagnosis, prevention strategies, and treatment are discussed in this article. Transfer metatarsalgia, recurrence, and hallux varus are discussed in Manuel Monteagudo and Pilar Martínez-de-Albornoz's article, "Management of Complications After Hallux Valgus Reconstruction," in this issue.

AVASCULAR NECROSIS OF THE FIRST METATARSAL HEAD

AVN of the first metatarsal head after metatarsal osteotomies is uncommon. Although spontaneous occurrence has been described,[9,10] it is more often presented as a complication of distal osteotomies in hallux valgus surgery. AVN also has been anecdotally reported with diaphyseal osteotomies such as a scarf, Ludloff, and Mao procedures.[11,12]

Historically, it was thought as a frequent complication of chevron osteotomy. This belief was based on a study by Meier and Kenzora in 1985 that reported 20% (12 of 60 feet) incidence of AVN with a chevron osteotomy and 50% (4 of 10 feet) when a lateral release was performed.[13] However, this high incidence of AVN has been contradicted by many other studies. Lee and colleagues[14] found no case of AVN in a series of 100 chevron osteotomies with lateral release. The same incidence was reported by Saro and colleagues[15] in 100 distal osteotomies.

Probably, the most important way to avoid this complication is to preserve the vascular anatomy of the metatarsal head during the surgery. For this purpose, a thorough understanding of vascular anatomy of the first metatarsal head is essential in hallux valgus surgery, as intraosseous blood supply to the metatarsal head is completely disrupted by the osteotomy.[16] The first metatarsal head is supplied by branches from the first dorsal metatarsal, first plantar metatarsal, and medial plantar arteries that create a plexus in the plantar lateral neck of the metatarsal (**Fig. 1**).

Jones and colleagues,[17] in 1995, studied the vascular supply of the metatarsal head in 22 specimens that underwent chevron osteotomy and lateral release. The investigators concluded with the following recommendations: the surgeon should avoid overpenetration of the lateral cortex with the saw along with extensive pericapsular stripping, the apex of the osteotomy should be at the center of the metatarsal head, and its plantar arm should exit the cortex proximal to the capsular insertion and distal to the nutrient artery.

Malal and colleagues[18] showed in a cadaveric study that the main vascular supply of the head is located in the plantar lateral corner of the metatarsal neck. In this study, they suggested that performing a chevron osteotomy with a long plantar limb exiting well proximal to the plantar capsule might decrease the risk of injury to the vessels and

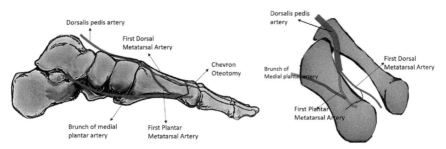

Fig. 1. First metatarsal head vascular supply by branches from the first dorsal metatarsal, first plantar metatarsal, and medial plantar arteries. Note that the first plantar metatarsal and the medial plantar artery create a plexus that enters in the lateral plantar neck of the metatarsal. To avoid AVN, the plantar arm should exit the cortex proximal to the capsular insertion and distal to the nutrient artery.

therefore may lessen the prevalence of osteonecrosis. Molloy and Widnall, in 2014, also recommended avoiding aggressive plantar dissection of the plantar neck at the level of capsular insertion because it is the only completely intact significant blood supply to the metatarsal head.[19]

Clinical presentation of AVN can vary greatly. Some patients are totally asymptomatic with slight radiographic changes and others can have devastating pain with advanced degenerative changes and bone collapse. The clinical findings can include pain, swelling, and stiffness of the MTP joint. Transfer metatarsalgia can also be found if the shortening of the first ray due to collapse of the metatarsal head has occurred.

Early radiographic findings include crescent-shaped subchondral lucencies, focal cyst formation, or mottling. Most of the time they disappear with the healing of the metatarsal osteotomy, as they only represent partial and restorable disturbance of the vascular supply. If AVN progresses, subchondral bony collapse, fragmentation of the head, and joint space narrowing can appear (**Fig. 2**). When AVN is suspected, an MRI is very specific for the diagnosis and can show the extent of head involvement.

Management depends on the degree of symptoms, deformity, and bone stock. Fortunately, most of the patients are asymptomatic or present with mild pain or stiffness and can be managed conservatively with a stiff soled shoe or an orthotic insole. Joint debridement, metaphyseal decompression, and bone marrow stimulation have been reported for early stages.[9] In severe cases, MTP arthrodesis is required. Interpositional structural bone graft must be used in the event when an important amount of necrotic bone has to be removed, to avoid transfer metatarsalgia caused by a short first ray.

NONUNION AND DELAYED UNION OF METATARSAL OSTEOTOMIES

Nonunion after metatarsal osteotomies is an uncommon complication. In a recent systematic review by Barg and colleagues,[4] including 7526 patients, the rate for nonunion was 0.04%. Half of the nonunions in this study were first tarsometatarsal (TMT) arthrodesis, so if we consider only the osteotomies, the nonunion rate is even lower. Proximal osteotomies are expected to have a higher rate of nonunion, as they have increased mechanical stress secondary to a bigger moment arm. Despite its infrequent rate, the treatment of this complication is challenging. For proper management of this condition, surgeons must differentiate when the nonunion is a result of a technical situation from a nonunion secondary to patient-related comorbidities.

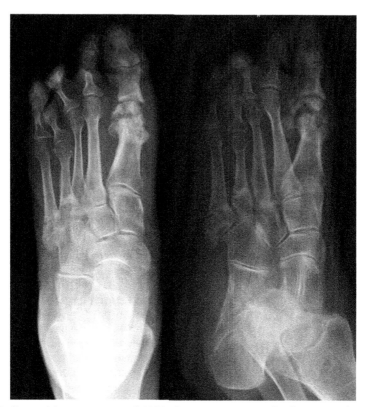

Fig. 2. Radiographic appearance of AVN after percutaneous distal metatarsal osteotomy performed in another hospital. The patient only had some stiffness and no pain.

Technical difficulties during surgery such as poorly performed osteotomies and inadequate fixation can result in delayed or nonunion. To prevent these problems it is important to consider general principles for osteotomies, including good surgical planning, protection of soft tissues (periosteum and joint capsule) to prevent damage to the bone blood supply, achievement of good surface contact prior fixation, and avoidance of bone thermal necrosis during the use of saws or burrs.[20]

Fixation method must be selected considering the bone mineral density of the patient and the inherent stability of the osteotomy. Surgeons must be aware of intraoperative incidents such as periimplant fractures (some of them very subtle) that may affect the stability of the fixation (**Fig. 3**). In this scenario, changing the position of screws or providing additional fixation can be necessary to achieve enough stability to assure bone healing.

Patient's related conditions that can affect bone healing must be considered before surgery. Factors such as nutritional status, compliance, bone mineral density, tobacco habit, medications, and comorbidities must be addressed and managed in order to prevent complications. Noncompliant patients with weight bearing are more likely to have fixation failures and potentially nonunion.[21] However, there is no consensus in the literature whether the early weight bearing can affect the outcomes of hallux valgus surgery. Vitamin D deficiency is particularly important, considering the high prevalence in the population. The prevalence of hypovitaminosis D in patients undergoing foot and ankle surgery is very high, with reported rates from 34% to 83%.[22–26] Although

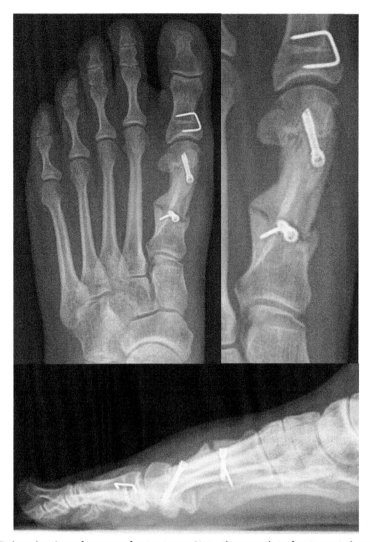

Fig. 3. Delayed union after a scarf osteotomy. Note the complete fracture at the proximal screw fixation site. Four months after initial surgery the bone healed. No additional procedures were needed.

we did not find any published evidence that correlated osteotomies for hallux valgus outcomes with vitamin D levels, a study compared 29 successful foot and ankle fusions with 29 nonunions. Statistical analysis revealed that patients with a preoperative diagnosis of vitamin D insufficiency or deficiency were 8 times more likely to develop a nonunion than patients who had sufficient vitamin D levels.[24] Because vitamin D supplementation is safe and the prevalence of hypovitaminosis is high, a routine preoperative check-up for vitamin D serum levels and supplementation is recommended when needed.

When suspected, computed tomographic (CT) bone scans can be useful to evaluate the consolidation status and to determine whether the bone healing process is active or not.

Conservative initial management of delayed unions and nonunion can be attempted, always considering the patient's condition and expectations. However, established nonunions are usually symptomatic and must be treated actively. In case of a bone healing delay, patient-related factors mentioned earlier must be checked and optimized. The use of bone stimulators has been helpful in the treatment of metatarsal nonunions secondary to trauma,[27] but its role in first metatarsal osteotomy has not been studied.[28]

Established and symptomatic nonunions, either due to no evolutive imaging or due to an inactive bone healing in CT scans, require surgical management to remove fibrous tissue and restore stability. Several factors must be considered before revision surgery. Once again, the authors emphasize the optimization of patient's modifiable factors that can affect bone healing. The location of the osteotomy and the remaining bone stock will dictate the necessity of bone grafting and the options of fixation. Large defects secondary to AVN or infection may require the use of structural bone block lengthening. Rigid and stable fixation with the use of locking plates is preferred, as the bone mineral density could be affected by the immobilization and low weight bearing. More distal or proximal locations with a poor bone stock, joints with severe damage and stiffness, and nonunions with severe deformities can require fusion of the adjacent joints to achieve stability.

MALUNION OF METATARSAL OSTEOTOMIES

Malunion is one of the most frequent causes of failure in hallux valgus surgery and can be defined as an improperly aligned and healed osteotomy. But when dealing with a complex deformity condition as hallux valgus, the achievement of a perfect restoration of alignment in all planes can be idealistic, and the limits to consider undercorrection or shortening as a malunion complication can be imprecise.

Every osteotomy has its own risk of specific malunion, and surgeons must know the intraoperative pitfalls to avoid this kind of complication. Most of the malunion cases have a deformity in multiple planes that need to be considered when planning treatment, but in order to organize the information about this topic, the authors describe each deformity separately.

Recurrence, iatrogenic varus, and transfer metatarsalgia are discussed in Manuel Monteagudo and Pilar Martínez-de-Albornoz's article, "Management of Complications," in this issue.

Shortening

Excluding opening wedge osteotomies, all metatarsal osteotomies generate some degree of shortening.

Several reports in the literature describe the extent of shortening of each osteotomy. In some of them, such as chevron and crescentic osteotomies, the expected shortening is only the width of the cutting saw (2–2.5 mm).[13] But others, such as biplanar chevron, Wilson, and Mitchell osteotomy, are expected to produce bigger shortening ranging from 3 to 7 mm.[29]

Shortening can be compensated by increasing the amount of plantar inclination of the longitudinal cut in a scarf osteotomy as the first metatarsal head can be slid to plantar (**Fig. 4**A, B).

Shortening of the first metatarsal can result in first ray insufficiency and transfer overload of central metatarsals during the third rocker. Symptoms will arise depending on the shortening magnitude and the relative length of the lesser metatarsals. The most common scenario associated with this kind of malunion is transfer metatarsalgia.

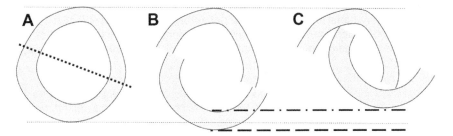

Fig. 4. (*A*) Obliquity of the osteotomy in the coronal plane determines the amount of plantar sliding of the head. Note the height difference (segmented *lines*) in the coronal plane between a well-performed oblique scarf (*B*) and troughing of the cortices (*C*).

Repetitive traumatic stress over the lesser metatarsals may damage the plantar plate, resulting in MP joint instability and stress fractures.[30,31]

The management of first ray insufficiency includes orthotics for mild cases. When planning surgical revision, restoration of a harmonic metatarsal parabola is of paramount importance. It can be achieved by first metatarsal lengthening, shortening of lesser metatarsals, or both.

Surgeons must be aware that lengthening can produce stiffness of first MTP joint caused by increased contact forces at MTP joint. Several techniques have been proposed for this purpose, such as lengthening scarf osteotomy, one-stage bone block distraction, and distraction osteogenesis with external fixation.[32,33] In cases of advanced arthritis of the first MTP joint, a bone block arthrodesis can be necessary.

Dorsal Malunion

Elevation of the metatarsal head can result after any osteotomy for hallux valgus correction but it is most frequently seen in proximal osteotomies (**Fig. 5**).

Dorsal malunions can affect severely the biomechanics of the forefoot. First metatarsal elevation can overload lesser metatarsal, and first MTP joint can go into plantar flexion causing interphalangeal joint dorsiflexion to restore the push-off function of the first toe. This kind of malunion may also cause restricted dorsiflexion of the MTP joint secondary to articular incongruence and dorsal impingement, leading to arthritis over time.

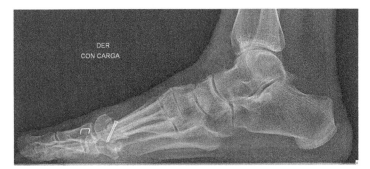

Fig. 5. An example of dorsal malunion after a chevron osteotomy. Note the orientation of the first metatarsal head. In this case, the probable cause of the complication was that the osteotomy was too distal in a poor-quality bone. At final follow-up, the patient was satisfied with the procedure and only an asymptomatic dorsal prominence was noticed.

The management of dorsal malunion depends on the severity of the residual deformity and the functional impairment of the patients. For mild cases, the use of an orthotic with a buildup beneath the first metatarsal head can be attempted. For more severe cases or failures after conservative treatment, well-planned revision surgery can be performed.

Several alternatives of osteotomies can be useful for this correction depending on the initial surgical technique, deformity in other planes, and the surgeon's preferences. A proximal dorsal opening wedge osteotomy using bone graft can plantarflex and restore length and varus of the first metatarsal. A crescentic proximal osteotomy is an alternative for uniplanar deformities and has the advantage of avoiding excessive shortening. Oblique osteotomies in the coronal plane such as chevron or scarf, to slide the head to a more plantar position, can restore the head positioning in 2 planes for selected patients (see **Fig. 4**A, B).

More complex deformities, with poor bone stock or instability/arthritis of first TMT joint, can be treated with a Lapidus arthrodesis. In this case, a plantar base bone wedge must be resected at the fusion level in order to plantarflex the first ray. Additional shortening procedures for lesser metatarsals should be evaluated when excessive shortening of the first metatarsal occurs after this technique. This technically challenging procedure has significantly higher rates of nonunion and should be reserved for selected cases.

Troughing

This type of malunion is specifically related to the scarf osteotomy and occurs when the cortices slide into the intramedullary canal of the proximal metatarsal shaft and lead to an elevation and loss of height of the distal segment (**Fig. 4**A, C). Troughing is a common complication for this procedure and has been reported in 35% of patients after scarf procedures[34] (**Fig. 6**) This complication can be associated with a rotational malunion due to supination of the distal segment when troughing occur.

Preventive strategies to avoid troughing have been described. Special attention must be paid in elderly patients with low bone density. Proximal and distal transverse cuts must be performed in metaphyseal bone, 10 to 15 mm from the joints. Interposition of resected cortical bone (or adductor hallucis tendon) into the intramedullary canal can be helpful to create compression without troughing. Also, temporary insertion

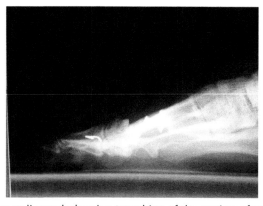

Fig. 6. Postoperative radiograph showing troughing of the cortices after a scarf osteotomy. The dorsal step observed at the level of distal osteotomy indicates the elevation of the first metatarsal head.

of a saw blade into the longitudinal cut before screw fixation has been described to avoid troughing.[35]

Plantarflexion Malunion

Plantarflexion deformity is an infrequent complication after hallux valgus surgery, because weight bearing usually tends to elevate the metatarsal head when a fixation failure occurs. This deformity is usually secondary to a technical intraoperative problem during deformity correction and fixation but also can be secondary to hardware failure.

Plantarflexion malunion leads to increased pressure under the first MTP joint and sesamoids, and symptoms can be aggravated in the context of dorsal impingement and hallux rigidus.

Nonsurgical treatment with orthotics with relief under the first MTP joint or Morton insoles can be attempted. Surgical options for treating this malunion include a dorsal closing wedge osteotomy or a proximal crescentic osteotomy (**Fig. 7**).

Isolated fusion of MTP joint is not enough to relieve the symptoms completely, as metatarsal-sesamoid articulation may persist overloaded. Patients with MTP arthritis may require a double procedure with an osteotomy to recover alignment and MTP fusion.

Rotational

Rotational malunions are complex and challenging deformities. Because of the supination of the first metatarsal commonly observed in hallux valgus, rotational malunion can be difficult to define as a complication. It is usually secondary to malreduction of the deformity intraoperatively.

Rotational deformities can affect the kinematics of the MTP joint and sesamoid complex, leading to restricted motion, pain, and, ultimately, degenerative arthritis.

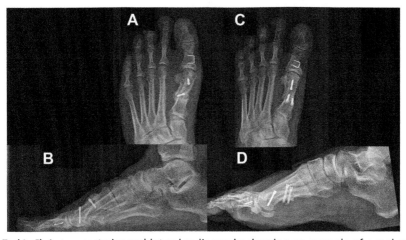

Fig. 7. (*A, B*) Anteroposterior and lateral radiographs showing an example of a malunited scarf osteotomy. The proximal screw was inserted too close to the proximal cut, causing a fracture. Varus and plantar flexion malunion can be seen. After remaining asymptomatic for 7 years, the patient presented with metatarsalgia of the first ray. (*C, D*) Dorsolateral base wedge osteotomy of the first metatarsal at the level of the malunion was performed and fixed with two 3.0-mm cannulated screws. Postoperative radiographs showing adequate correction of the deformity.

This type of deformity is difficult to study. Weight-bearing CT should give the best information, but because its availability is scarce, other imaging studies such as the axial sesamoid view, CT, or single-photon emission computerized tomography-CT could help to objectivate the metatarsal rotation (**Fig. 8**).

Attempts of conservative management are rarely successful, as orthotic management cannot adequately correct the deformity. Surgical management is challenging due to the necessity of correction of a multiplanar deformity. Osteotomies that allow derotation of the metatarsal must be selected. Usually, the intrinsic stability of the osteotomy is lost, and more stable fixation and bone graft may be needed.

Fusion of the MTP joint is reserved for cases with severe degenerative changes, but for cases of complex deformity and stiffness, a fusion can be a more predictable treatment option.

METATARSOPHALANGEAL ARTHRITIS

The incidence of MTP osteoarthritis after osteotomies for hallux valgus correction is not usually reported. Because most of the patients with hallux valgus have some articular incongruence preoperative, it is difficult to know whether degenerative changes found after surgery are caused by the surgery itself or is a consequence of the preoperative deformity and joint damage.

Logically thinking, if a preoperative articular incongruence is well corrected with hallux valgus surgery, one should expect that the biomechanical conditions of the joint are improved, and degenerative changes should not appear or progress. However, most of the complications discussed previously in this article can lead to degenerative changes at the MTP joint.

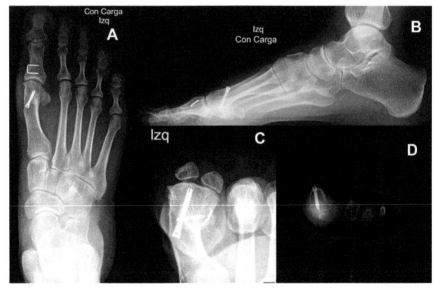

Fig. 8. Example of a rotational malunion. The patient complaint was plantar pain localized at the sesamoids. (*A*) and (*B*) show an acceptable correction of intermetatarsal angle, but the sesamoids were not centered. (*C*) Axial view of sesamoids showing the rotation of the metatarsal head. (*D*) SPECT-CT of the same case showing an increased uptake at the sesamoids due to malrotation.

Degenerative changes in first MTP joint after hallux valgus surgery can arise from AVN of first metatarsal head, leading to cartilage damage or articular incongruence and increased contact forces at MTP joint level after metatarsal malunion.

As discussed previously, vascular injury to the metatarsal head can progress to chondrolysis and advanced osteoarthritis. Aggressive dissection during surgery, especially around the metatarsal neck, can damage the arterial supply. Also, when a distal osteotomy is performed, such as a chevron, the plantar cut must end proximal to the metatarsal neck in order to keep the blood supply through the plantar metatarsal artery.[36]

Conflicting evidence exists about the cause of hallux rigidus. Coughlin and Shurmas in 2003 showed, in 110 patients surgically treated for hallux rigidus, no association with first metatarsal elevation, gastrocnemius or Achilles contracture, and long first metatarsal.[37] On the other hand, there are several clinical and biomechanical studies that show good results with decompressive, shortening, or plantarflexion osteotomies for hallux rigidus.[38,39] Plantar fascia contracture also has been found related to hallux rigidus or limitus.[40,41]

According to this evidence, hallux rigidus could develop after metatarsal osteotomies when they heal in dorsiflexion or when the metatarsal is lengthened. As discussed previously, troughing, stress fracture, or fixation failure can lead to metatarsal dorsiflexion. Proximal opening wedge osteotomies theoretically could increase contact pressure at MTP joint; however, Kia and colleagues,[42] in 2017, showed no statistical significance in MTP contact pressure between specimens with hallux valgus after proximal opening wedge osteotomy, scarf osteotomy, and with no osteotomy.

In asymptomatic patients with MTP arthritis after hallux valgus surgery, only clinical observation is recommended.

In symptomatic patients who do not respond to conservative management after at least 6 months, surgery is indicated.

When only dorsiflexion pain at the extreme range of motion is found and radiologically the main finding is a dorsal spur with no significant malalignment, a cheilectomy is suggested.

In cases with moderate cartilage damage where evident dorsal deviation and elevation of the first metatarsal is observed, our treatment is a decompressive metatarsal osteotomy. Our preferred method is the Youngswick osteotomy. This modification of the chevron osteotomy allows shortening and/or plantar flexion of the first ray.[43] For severe arthritis with midrange pain, an MTP fusion is performed.

SUMMARY

Most of the complications of hallux valgus surgery can be prevented with proper surgical planning and a careful surgical technique.

Metatarsal head AVN and nonunion are very infrequent complications following metatarsal osteotomies.

Intrinsic stability and location of the osteotomy, type of fixation, careful anatomic dissection, and comorbidities, including vitamin D deficiency and bone quality, can influence the occurrence of these complications.

Shortening, elevation, plantarflexion, varus/valgus, and rotational are the most common deformities that need to be considered when planning treatment of a malunion.

MTP osteoarthritis can develop after metatarsal malunion or AVN. Treatment options include cheilectomy, osteotomies to correct malunions, and MTP arthrodesis.

DISCLOSURE

The authors have nothing to disclose.

REFERENCES

1. Nix S, Smith M, Vicenzino B. Prevalence of Hallux Valgus in the general population: a systematic review and meta-analysis. J Foot Ankle Res 2010. https://doi.org/10.1186/1757-1146-3-21.
2. Jeuken RM, Schotanus MGM, Kort NP, et al. Long-term follow-up of a randomized controlled trial comparing scarf to chevron osteotomy in hallux valgus correction. Foot Ankle Int 2016;37(7):687–95.
3. Bock P, Kluger R, Kristen KH. The Scarf Osteotomy with minimally invasive lateral release for treatment of hallux valgus deformity. J Bone Joint Surg Am 2015;97(15):1238–45.
4. Barg A, Harmer JR, Presson AP, et al. Unfavorable outcomes following surgical treatment of hallux valgus deformity. J Bone Joint Surg 2018;100(18):1563–73.
5. Vora AM, Myerson MS. First metatarsal osteotomy nonunion and malunion. Foot Ankle Clin 2005;10(1):35–54.
6. Raikin SM, Miller AG, Daniel J. Recurrence of hallux valgus: a review. Foot Ankle Clin 2014;19(2):260–74.
7. Schuh R, Willegger M, Holinka J, et al. Angular correction and complications of proximal first metatarsal osteotomies for hallux valgus deformity. Int Orthop 2013;37(9):1771–80.
8. Cody EA, Foot O, Surgery A, et al. Influence of diagnosis and other factors on patients' expectations of foot and ankle surgery. Foot Ankle Int 2018;39(6):641–8.
9. Fu FH, Gomez W. Bilateral avascular necrosis of the first metatarsal head in adolescence. A case report. Clin Orthop Relat Res 1989;246:282–4.
10. Suzuki J, Tanaka Y, Omokawa S, et al. Idiopathic osteonecrosis of the first metatarsal head: a case report. Clin Orthop Relat Res 2003;415(415):239–43.
11. Easley ME, Kelly IP. Avascular necrosis of the hallux metatarsal head. Foot Ankle Clin 2000;5(3):591–608.
12. Wallace GF, Bellacosa R, Mancuso JE. Avascular necrosis following distal first metatarsal osteotomies: a survey. J Foot Ankle Surg 1994;33(2):167–72.
13. Meier PJ, Kenzora JE. The risks and benefits of distal first metatarsal osteotomies. Foot Ankle 1985;6(1):7–17.
14. Lee KB, Cho NY, Park HW, et al. A comparison of proximal and distal Chevron osteotomy, both with lateral soft-tissue release, for moderate to severe hallux valgus in patients undergoing simultaneous bilateral correction: a prospective randomised controlled trial. Bone Joint J 2015;97-B(2):202–7.
15. Saro C, Andrén B, Wildemyr Z, et al. Outcome after distal metatarsal osteotomy for hallux valgus: a prospective randomized controlled trial of two methods. Foot Ankle Int 2007;28(7):778–87.
16. Gurevich M, Bialik V, Eidelman M, et al. Avascular necrosis of the 1st metatarsal head. Acta Chir Orthop Traumatol Cech 2008;75(5):396–8.
17. Jones KJ, Feiwell LA, Freedman EL, et al. The effect of chevron osteotomy with lateral capsular release on the blood supply to the first metatarsal head. J Bone Joint Surg Am 1995;77(2):197–204.
18. Malal JJG, Shaw-Dunn J, Kumar CS, et al. Blood supply to the first metatarsal head and vessels at risk with a chevron osteotomy. J Bone Joint Surg Am 2007;89(9):2018–22.
19. Molloy A, Widnall J. Scarf osteotomy. Foot Ankle Clin 2014;19:165–80.

20. Baravarian B, Ben-Ad R. Revision hallux valgus. Causes and correction options. Clin Podiatr Med Surg 2014;31(2):291–8.
21. Campbell B, Schimoler P, Belagaje S, et al. Weight-bearing recommendations after first metatarsophalangeal joint arthrodesis fixation: a biomechanical comparison. J Orthop Surg Res 2017;12(1):23.
22. Bogunovic L, Kim AD, Beamer BS, et al. Hypovitaminosis D in patients scheduled to undergo orthopaedic surgery: a single-center analysis. J Bone Joint Surg Am 2010;92(13):2300–4.
23. Michelson JD, Charlson MD. Vitamin D status in an elective orthopedic surgical population. Foot Ankle Int 2016;37(2):186–91.
24. Moore KR, Howell MA, Saltrick KR, et al. Risk factors associated with nonunion after elective foot and ankle reconstruction: a case-control study. J Foot Ankle Surg 2017;56(3):457–62.
25. Aujla RS, Allen PE, Ribbans WJ. Vitamin D levels in 577 consecutive elective foot & ankle surgery patients. Foot Ankle Surg 2017. https://doi.org/10.1016/J.FAS.2017.12.007.
26. DeFontes K, Smith JT. Surgical considerations for Vitamin D deficiency in foot and ankle surgery. Orthop Clin North Am 2019;50(2):259–67.
27. Nolte PA, van der Krans A, Patka P, et al. Low-intensity pulsed ultrasound in the treatment of nonunions. J Trauma 2001;51(4):693–702 [discussion: 702–3].
28. Becker A. First metatarsal malunion. Foot Ankle Clin 2009;14(1):77–90.
29. Lee KT, Park YU, Jegal H, et al. Deceptions in hallux valgus. Foot Ankle Clin 2014; 19(3):361–70.
30. Goldberg A, Singh D. Treatment of shortening following hallux valgus surgery. Foot Ankle Clin 2014;19(2):310–6.
31. Maceira E, Monteagudo M. Transfer metatarsalgia post hallux valgus surgery. Foot Ankle Clin 2014;19(2):286–307.
32. Hurst JM, Nunley JA. Distraction osteogenesis for the shortened metatarsal after hallux valgus surgery. Foot Ankle Int 2007;28(2):194–8.
33. Bevilacqua NJ, Rogers LC, Wrobel JS, et al. Restoration and preservation of first metatarsal length using the distraction scarf osteotomy. J Foot Ankle Surg 2008; 47(2):96–102.
34. Coetzee JC. Scarf osteotomy for Hallux valgus repair: the dark side. Foot Ankle Int 2003;24(1):29–33.
35. Lee SC, Hwang SH, Nam CH, et al. Technique for preventing troughing in scarf osteotomy. J Foot Ankle Surg 2017;56(4):822–3.
36. Rothwell M, Pickard J. The chevron osteotomy and avascular necrosis. Foot 2013;23:34–8.
37. Coughlin MJ, Shurnas PS. Hallux Rigidus grading and long-term results of operative treatment. J Bone Joint Surg Am 2003. https://doi.org/10.1097/BTF.0b013e318254aa0d.
38. Derner R, Goss K, Noel Postowski H, et al. A plantarflexory-shortening osteotomy for hallux rigidus: a retrospective analysis. J Foot Ankle Surg 2005;44(5):377–89.
39. Migues A, Slullitel G. Joint-preserving procedure for moderate hallux rigidus. Foot Ankle Clin 2012. https://doi.org/10.1016/j.fcl.2012.06.006.
40. Flavin R, Halpin T, O'sullivan R, et al. A finite-element analysis study of the metatarsophalangeal joint of the hallux rigidus. J Bone Joint Surg Br 2008;90(10): 1334–40.
41. Viehöfer AF, Vich M, Wirth SH, et al. The role of plantar fascia tightness in hallux limitus: a biomechanical analysis. J Foot Ankle Surg 2019. https://doi.org/10.1053/j.jfas.2018.09.019.

42. Kia C, Yoshida R, Cote M, et al. First metatarsophalangeal contact properties following proximal opening wedge and scarf osteotomies for hallux valgus correction: a biomechanical study. Foot Ankle Int 2017;38(4):430–5.

43. Youngswick FD. Modifications of the Austin bunionectomy for treatment of metatarsus primus elevatus associated with hallux limitus. J Foot Surg 1982;21(2):114–6.

Moving?

Make sure your subscription moves with you!

To notify us of your new address, find your **Clinics Account Number** (located on your mailing label above your name), and contact customer service at:

Email: journalscustomerservice-usa@elsevier.com

800-654-2452 (subscribers in the U.S. & Canada)
314-447-8871 (subscribers outside of the U.S. & Canada)

Fax number: 314-447-8029

Elsevier Health Sciences Division
Subscription Customer Service
3251 Riverport Lane
Maryland Heights, MO 63043

Printed and bound by CPI Group (UK) Ltd, Croydon, CR0 4YY

03/10/2024

01040483-0018